Doing Disney
on a Special Diet

*All Natural Mom's Guide to Avoiding Dyes, Artificial
Flavors, and Other Food Allergens While Enjoying the Parks*

By Sheri Davis

Acknowledgments

I would like to thank Walt Disney for never giving up on his dream and creating such a phenomenal theme park! It truly *is* the happiest place on earth!

I would also like to thank my kids, Cody, Lynsey, Dylan, and Brooklyn for giving me a reason to go to Disney so many times!

And thank you to my Lord and Savior for the many blessings you have bestowed upon me and my family.

Soli Deo Gloria.

Dedicated to my parents, Ron and Jean Williamson who made it possible for me to take my kids to Disney more times than I can count. Thank you!

Contents

Introduction

I love Disney! We used to go every year so it can be done when avoiding the Big 3, (which I refer to as dyes, artificial flavors, and the preservatives BHT, BHA, and TBHQ), or if you're dealing with other food allergies. We've had lots of practice so I'll share what we do.

I should probably first introduce myself. I am the author of *"All Natural Mom's Guide to the Feingold Diet - A Natural Approach to ADHD and Other Related Disorders."* I have four kids ages 16, 13, 10, and 6; two boys and two girls. We have dealt with and overcome symptoms of ADHD, high functioning autism, Lyme disease, dyslexia, seizures, and food allergies.

Our family follows the Feingold Diet as our foundation. For the first few years on the Feingold Diet, we limited foods high in salicylates, but we have been able to add them back into our diet in moderation. My three youngest and myself follow a gluten and dairy free (GFCF) diet in addition to Feingold. My oldest does Feingold only with limited dairy.

If you avoid dyes or other additives but aren't familiar with the Feingold Diet, I of course highly suggest you read my first book or visit my blog at www.allnaturalmomof4.com. You can also find helpful information on Feingold's web site at www.feingold.org.

For a short run-down - the Feingold Diet is best known as an ADHD diet, though it is helpful for many other issues as well. The concepts of the Feingold Diet are beneficial for anyone who eats.

There are two stages to the diet. In stage one, you will avoid both the Big 3 (dyes, artificial flavors, and preservatives), and foods high in salicylates (sals). Salicylates are the natural chemicals that plants produce to ward off bugs and diseases - think natural pesticide. [1]

Some people lack the necessary enzymes (the PST enzymes specifically) to break down and process these natural substances (the salicylates), causing a physical and/or behavioral reaction. Kids or adults with ADHD are often low in this enzyme, which is why the Feingold Diet is often very helpful for them.

In our case, my son who was four at the time was a completely different child within two days of removing both the Big 3 and foods high in salicylates. Almost all of his ADHD symptoms disappeared as long as he stayed on diet. We were eventually able to add back in foods high in salicylates and move to stage two of the diet, where you only avoid the Big 3. Many people still limit the amount of salicylates in their diets though, and we do as well.

Whether you just avoid the Big 3, or your child also avoids other food groups as well and you're headed to Disney, this guide is a great resource. There's a lot of information that can be helpful to know ahead of time to make your vacation more enjoyable for everyone.

And obviously, I can't cover every single food allergen specifically so I've written about our own family's experiences at Disney. Use your best judgement in deciding how to handle your family's specific food allergies and preferences.

If you are new to eating gluten and dairy free, please familiarize yourself with those foods that are free of gluten and dairy. I mention foods throughout the book that my older son eats that are not GFCF, but are free of the Big 3.

I originally had this information as a chapter in my next book, *"Living Dye Free in a Cotton Candy World - All Natural Mom's Guide to Avoiding Dyes, Artificial Flavors, and Preservatives in Every Day Life for Happier, Healthier Kids"* but decided to make it a short stand-alone book instead as it started to take on a life of its own!

If you are new to special diets, this information may feel overwhelming at first, but it gets easier each time you plan a vacation and it's really worth it when you can have a nice, peaceful vacation without meltdowns or reactions. Planning ahead is absolutely essential.

There have been a few isolated times where I thought, "I'm not gonna worry about the food. We're on vacation." I have regretted it every single time. Why? Because instead of taking a little extra time to plan, I had to deal with kids who were reacting, which put a damper on our vacation.

I'd much rather worry about the food than deal with the repercussions of crabby, hyper, fighting, crying, or sick kids afterward. That's not to say that we are always 100% on diet while on vacation. When you're not at home, some things are out of your control like cross-contamination issues or unexpected events, but we certainly do our best.

Many of the ideas presented in this book also apply to vacationing just about anywhere. I've only taken my kids to Disney World in

Orlando, Florida so I reference Orlando specifically but most of this information will apply to Disneyland in California as well.

There are references to both flying to Disney or driving, and staying at a condo with a full kitchen, or staying in a regular hotel room. While you won't be doing both, you may be doing each of these at different times for different vacations, so you may find the information helpful for other times.

After reading this book, I hope you'll feel more confident and at peace shouting, "Hey kids! We're going to Disney World!" But most of all, I hope this guide will help you make the most of your trip to the happiest place on earth and make some beautiful family memories!

Chapter 1
Meal Planning

The number one rule when you have a child on a special diet is: Be prepared! Whether you'll have a full kitchen or not, I recommend making a meal plan before you leave for vacation along with a shopping list for groceries. I hate making meal plans because it takes so much time, but trust me, it's worth it! You'll be glad you did.

If at any time I start to feel lazy and think, "Ugh, we'll just wing it this time." I remind myself of what happened at Magic Kingdom a few years ago. One of my kids refused to eat the sandwich I packed him for dinner. He had been on a clean diet for several years and wasn't as sensitive to eating off diet as my other kids. He really wanted to eat at the park and he also wanted ice cream, which he typically avoids because of a dairy sensitivity.

I reluctantly let him go off with his grandpa and he got a big chocolate soft serve ice cream cone. For dinner, he had a BBQ pulled pork sandwich from the park (which probably had dyes in the BBQ sauce and who knows what else).

By the time we were leaving the park, he started saying his stomach hurt and he didn't feel good. Waiting in line for the tram to take us back to our car in the parking lot, he was on the ground, crying, barely able to walk. He was too old to sit in the stroller, so he managed to make it back to the car.

As soon as we pulled in to our parking space at our condo, he threw up all over our rental minivan. After getting the rest of the kids into our room and settled, I went back to clean up the van. And at that point, I thought to myself, I think I'll listen to the whining next time instead of giving in and letting him eat irresponsibly. It's not worth the mess I'll have to deal with after!

I do have a chapter on how to make the best choices if you choose to eat at the park, but your best bet is to bring your own food or plan your meals carefully, knowing what your safest options are.

When you have a meal plan, you can bring what you need from home, and you'll know exactly what you need from the store when you get there. And the next time you go on vacation, you can work from this same meal plan if you'd like. (See the end of this book for a sample meal plan and shopping list to help you get started.)

When we first started avoiding the Big 3, I never made a meal plan and just went shopping when I got to Florida. Big mistake. We wasted so much food and had to throw out a lot the day we left, which means we wasted a lot of money as well. Since we typically stay at a place close to Whole Foods, I now get what I think we'll need for the first half of the week and then go back for more groceries later in the week.

When making your meal plan, also make a list of things you can bring from home as well like spices. I bring taco seasoning, hamburger seasoning, chicken nugget "breading", sea salt, etc. Don't forget to bring along any recipes you'll need as well.

If we're only having rice one night, I'll measure out how much rice we need and pack it in my suitcase. I do the same with cereal. You could also buy these items when you get there but sometimes you don't know what the stores will have in stock and if I know only one of my kids is going to eat one kind of cereal one day, I'd rather bring one serving than buy a whole box. I'll also bring along any other snacks that can be hard to find in stores.

I also pack any other miscellaneous items we might need like sippy cups, refillable insulated water bottles for the parks, Tupperware for fruit and sandwiches, a ceramic bowl and spoons for cereal and oatmeal, insulated food thermoses, zip lock bags, enzymes, vitamins, probiotics, etc. (See the end of this book for a full list of suggested items to bring).

Shipping Your Food

When flying, some people go so far as to pack an entire suitcase with food. While I have packed a few food items in my suitcase, I've never filled an entire suitcase. If you get free luggage with your airline, this can be economical. However, if you have to pay for luggage, you could be paying up to $70 to bring your food with you.

And remember you'll have to pay for shipping both ways unless you pack the food in a collapsible bag that you can pack in another suitcase on the way back. I usually try to pack as much food as I can in our carry-on backpacks.

Another option is to ship a box of food to your hotel or condo ahead of time. Call ahead to find out what your hotel's policy is and how you should address the box. Try to ship it so it gets there a couple of days before you arrive. Most places will hold the box for you until you arrive. A select few of the Disney hotels will charge a fee for doing this. Shipping charges will vary of course depending on how heavy and big the box is.

Another option for shipping your food is using Amazon Prime Pantry. [2] They currently charge $5.99 per box. I have not personally used this service before. The only drawback is the limited availability since you would only be shipping dry goods. If you are staying at a family member's house, I would just order on Amazon as usual and ship to my family's address, making sure the food arrives before I get there.

Groceries Delivered

If you don't have a car, you can have your groceries delivered to your hotel or condo. This also saves you time. I have not personally used these services but a lot of families with food allergies have. Here are the top three recommended grocery services. For updated info on pricing and options, visit their web sites.

1. Garden Grocer - 866-855-4350 - www.gardengrocer.com

Call or order ahead of time (at least a week is preferable but there is a 36-hour minimum) and choose your delivery date and time (you get a two hour window). Discounts are given the earlier you place your order so plan ahead. You can get up to 10% off by ordering 60 days in advance which is highly recommended.

You can call and talk to someone if you have any questions and then you will place your order online. They have a large selection of brands to choose from but they don't list foods by specific stores. You can do a search at the top of their web site for the items on your list.

Fees: Currently the delivery fee is $14 for orders totaling between $40 to $200. You must order a minimum of $40 in groceries. Grocery bills over $200 have a delivery fee of only $2. [1]

2. WeGoShop - 877-934-6746 - www.wegoshop.com

This service is similar to Garden Grocer but they will go to multiple stores which is nice if you need things from both Whole Foods and Publix or Trader Joe's. Their fees are a little higher though.

Fees: Currently the delivery fee is between $24-$29 for orders between $50 to $200, and an additional $5 for each additional store. They also add an extra 10% for gratuity if the groceries will be dropped off at the hotel's front desk. [2]

3. Whole Foods - 407-355-7100 - www.wholefoodsmarket.com

Whole Foods will deliver groceries to most Disney hotels. Call ahead to confirm. Then go to Whole Foods' web site and click on the "Grocery Delivery" button and type in the zip code where you will be staying. As an example, the Disney Port Orleans Resort zip code is 32830. They request at least a 48-hour notice and they'll add a 10% gratuity to your bill.

Fees: Fees are based on how far away your hotel is. It can range anywhere from $20 to $80. Disney hotels are currently listed at $30.

Keep in mind you will also want to tip your delivery person. Certain hotels like the Swan and Dolphin (not owned by Disney but on Disney's property on the Boardwalk) do not accept grocery deliveries. Disney's Beach and Yacht Club only accept deliveries at a set time each day which is currently between 4:30pm and 5:30pm.

Using Uber or Taxis

Your other option is to use Uber or taxi services to go grocery shopping yourself. Maybe I'm a control freak, but I personally like to do my own grocery shopping. I don't trust the kind of produce someone else might pick out! There are lots of Uber drivers in Orlando so it shouldn't be a problem to take one to the store and then call another one when you're done shopping, and some drivers will wait while you shop. Just ask.

You can also use Uber during your stay to get to any restaurants. If you're staying at a Disney hotel, you can also use the Disney bus transportation system to get to any other Disney hotels or to Disney Springs (formerly Downtown Disney) if you plan on eating at those places.

If you've never used Uber before, look online for a code for first-time users. You can get your first ride free (up to a $15 value). And for tips on how to use Uber at Disney, check out this informative article: http://www.disneytouristblog.com/uber-disney-world-tips/. [3]

Rent a Car

This is the only way we vacation. I like the convenience of having a car and being able to run to the store whenever I need to. It does add to the cost of your vacation but hey, you're at Disney. You're already spending a boat load. Don't forget the car seat if you have a little one and I always bring my car charger for my cell phone. Just don't forget it in the car when you go back home! I did that once.

If you have a car, there are lots of options for shopping. There is a Whole Foods at 8003 Turkey Lake Road, near International Drive and Sea World. We stayed at Disney's Port Orleans this summer and it was about a 15 to 20 minute drive, depending on traffic.

There is a Wal-Mart right across the street from Whole Foods that has a full grocery department. Publix is a good option for a regular grocery store as well. There is one just down the street from Whole Foods at 7640 Sand Lake Road.

Keep going down the street from Publix and you'll hit the Trader Joe's at 8323 Sand Lake Road. And if you need a health food store, Chamberlin's Natural Foods is at 7600 Dr. Phillips Blvd. which is right in that same area. There's also a Five Guy's Restaurant in that same shopping center. Bonus! (These addresses are listed again in chapter 10 under Resources.)

Sometimes even with a meal plan though, plans can change. Whatever food we have leftover that we haven't opened, I try to return on the last day so I save my receipts.

Driving to Disney

If you're close enough and able to drive to Orlando, you can load up your car with a big old cooler and bring all your own food! Yay! Or stop at a grocery store when you get there. My mom lives three hours from Orlando during the winter, so she would meet us in Orlando. She made a few things at her house beforehand and brought them up with her. Things like pancakes, muffins, chicken nuggets, chili, stew, etc. Then she just threw it in the freezer when she got there. That way, we didn't have to spend as much of our time on vacation cooking. We just heated up the food. That was really nice.

Chapter 2
The Airport

If you're flying to Disney, you'll need to plan what you're going to bring on the plane for snacks for both ways. When we fly to Florida, we always miss a meal so that needs to be packed as well. I try to pack what I can the night before as the morning is usually super busy. I usually pack cut up fruit, sandwiches, turkey rolls, or summer sausage and crackers.

Airports generally don't want you to travel with any liquids but I have passed through security with chili, chicken stew, and spaghetti in a thermos. I wouldn't try to get through with soup though. They would just test the food in our thermos (by holding a little strip over it) and tell us not to bring any "liquids" next time. I always just tell the security person that my kids have allergies.

I try to be nice, and giving them my best "It's been a really long morning and I have four kids and lots of luggage in tow so if you'd be so nice as to just let us through as quickly as possible, I'd really appreciate it." look always helps. If you want to take it a step further, you could get your doctor to write you a note and flash it at them.

It's against HIPAA laws for them to ask for specifics about your child's medical diagnosis, but your doctor can write a general letter stating that due to medical reasons, your children need to bring their own food from home when traveling. [1] I've never done this because we've always passed through security without any problems. I try to be as nice as possible with the security personnel though. I think that helps and honestly, I think they just feel sorry for me travelling with so many kids and they just pass us along!

A lot of times now we are already TSA pre-approved. That's always nice. They just randomly do that for some people when they feel you are not a threat. We didn't have to wait in a long line and they didn't check our bags as thoroughly. I think they just heard about all the crap we bring and they didn't want us to hold up the lines!

I've made it through with lemonade in a sippy cup or sports bottle as well. I tell them it has my kids' supplements in it which it always does. They just test it. You can also bring a cooler type bag as well as long as you have some supplements/medication in it. I put our probiotics in it. That way we can keep some of our food cold too.

I pack an ice brick, not a bag of ice as the ice will melt and be considered a liquid that they will ask you to throw out. Or you can just empty your bag of ice when you get to the airport before going through security. After going through security, stop at a restaurant like McDonald's and ask for a cup of ice to refill your zip lock bag.

I have a cooler backpack that I purchased online. It's great for travelling and bringing to the parks. We use it all the time. The only down side is that it isn't very big so it doesn't hold a ton but it's handy. They will often check your bag when you have food in it, so don't be surprised. They're just doing their jobs.

Now I take my thermos out of the backpack and put it up on the conveyor belt separately because apparently it looks like a bomb! Otherwise, they always have to check the whole bag.

If you don't want to go through the x-ray detector (to avoid radiation) you can ask to be searched manually. I've been pulled out of line for a random check before. It's not a big deal. They just pat you down.

Operation Distract the Kids

As a side note, to keep your kids entertained during the flight, always bring things to keep them busy. For young toddlers, new stickers were always a hit with my kids. I brought a ton and just kept handing my toddler stickers one at a time to stick on paper or a coloring book.

Other ideas include playing cards, new DS games, new apps or movies for their iPads, new travel games, new coloring books and markers, or new books - the key word here being "new." Do not under any circumstances let them see or give them these things before you are seated on the plane. After take-off is the best time to break out your stash of goodies as they'll be distracted for the first twenty minutes by the newness of being on the plane.

Also, always determine ahead of time who will sit in the window seat! We take turns with who gets the seat going down and coming back. If we have 3 kids vying for a seat, the youngest gets priority as my older ones have flown more in their lifetime. If you wait until you get on the plane to decide, expect World War III (I speak from experience).

If you're relying on the iPads to keep the kids entertained, don't forget that you have to turn these off during take-off and landing. Toddlers don't understand this concept and will cry bloody murder if you take away their electronics after they've started doing something on it.

And don't forget headphones for *each* child. Our last flight had TV screens on the back of each seat and you could choose which movie you wanted to watch. They had a bunch of new movies too. My kids loved it! But, you need headphones to be able to watch/hear the movie.

I've also bribed my kids with money. I give them each a certain amount of money as spending money for the trip. When they were little, I'd give them a roll of quarters. My boys equated coins with game room money. If they didn't behave, they would lose a quarter.

Food at the Airport

Snacks can also keep the kids occupied for a short time. This year for snacks on the plane, I brought my girls some Boom Chicka Pop popcorn, Whole Foods 365 beef jerky, B-Fresh and Glee bubble gum, and some Surf Sweet peach gummy rings as a treat or in place of the gum for take-off.

I brought myself some dried fruit. I make bananas, apples, pears, pineapple, or kale chips in my dehydrator ahead of time. I try to make it at least a week in advance so I'm not making everything the day before we leave. I also like to bring a Nugo GFCF chocolate pretzel protein bar or a Kind maple glazed pecan and sea salt bar. After we go through security, we sometimes buy an individual serving size of Simply Lemonade and Fiji water.

You never know when your flight might get delayed. Living in Chicago, our flight has been delayed more times than I'd like to remember in the winter. Not fun. Always be prepared.

These days, there always seems to be at least one airport store that sells healthier options like fresh fruit and a few clean snacks. Just expect to pay a lot of money for those snacks! That's why I try to pack as much food as we can in our backpacks.

A couple of airports have Aunt Annie's soft pretzels. My son gets a plain pretzel with salt and butter or a cinnamon sugar pretzel, and their lemonade. Mrs. Field's chocolate chip cookies are also currently free of the Big 3. The prepackaged Mrs. Field's cookies are not; only the cookies made fresh at the stores.

If we absolutely have to eat at the airport, we'll usually opt for McDonald's or Wendy's. See chapter 5 for more details on what we order when eating out.

At the Orlando airport there is a McDonald's and Auntie Anne's pretzels before you go through security, and there is a Wendy's after security near the gates.

Lay's potato chips or Fritos are snacks that my kids like that we can usually find anywhere. Wait, I feed my family Lay's? Yes. Yes, I do. Please don't send me e-mails. Lay's potato chips and Fritos used to be acceptable on Feingold before Lay's decided to stop filling out forms. As far as I know, ingredients have not changed and I believe they are still free of the Big 3. We only eat them on occasion.

Pringles Original is another option free of the Big 3 but they do contain gluten and corn syrup if you avoid those ingredients. While these are not the healthiest options, when we're on vacation, we do the best we can and try not to sweat the small stuff. All things in moderation as well. Choose snacks and foods based on your family's preferences and needs.

Random Tip

Before leaving the house for vacation, I usually leave a few cotton balls dipped in olive oil with a few drops of peppermint oil and leave them in areas where we sometimes get ants. If you soak the cotton balls in water only, the water will evaporate faster than the oil.

Ants hate peppermint (as do spiders and mice). I forgot to do this on our last trip and we came home to a large gathering of ants near the front door and in my kitchen sink! Note to self: Next time take a later flight so I have time to put away the dirty dishes I made preparing breakfast and lunch.

I also have a homemade ant killer spray I make that I'll spray in the areas the ants we get like to travel. They know their way to my kitchen! I've sprayed this on forming bee hives as well and the bees never came back to the hive. (Recipe at the end of this book.)

Chapter 3
Accommodations with a Full Kitchen

There are two ways to do Disney on a special diet - stay in a regular hotel room or stay at a hotel or condo/house with a full kitchen. I always recommend trying to stay somewhere *with* a full kitchen. Having a full kitchen makes it much easier to keep your kids on a special diet, and you might be surprised that the price difference for getting a room with a full kitchen is not always that much more expensive.

My guess is the hotels may not have as much demand for full kitchens so they don't charge a whole lot more. The money you'll save by not eating out as much is going to more than pay for the difference in price for accommodations with a full kitchen.

If you have a large family (6 or more), you probably already know that sometimes the hotel forces you to get two rooms. When you have to pay for more than one room, it often becomes cheaper to rent a two bedroom villa, which usually comes with a full kitchen.

Timeshares

My parents happen to own a timeshare in Orlando, Florida at Westgate Lakes which is right across the street from a Whole Foods and minutes from several clean restaurants and a health food store.

Huge plus! Westgate is right by SeaWorld and about 10 to 15 minutes from the Disney parks.

Many timeshares offer a greatly reduced rate if you stay with them and listen to a one or two hour speech and tour of their grounds. We did that at another Westgate location near Branson, Missouri once and only paid $50 a night for our room.

So, that's another option if you can hold your ground and not buy, but do your research first. My parents don't think the timeshare was worth the money but they can afford it so they keep it for the grandkids.

Disney has their own timeshares as well but they are very expensive. We went to one of their timeshare pitches this past year and got a free $100 Disney gift card for listening to their sales person for about an hour. We had received a coupon for the gift card in our Disney hotel room. It was raining and we had nothing else to do. Warning: They give out cupcakes but they have some Enjoy Life cookies for those with allergies. Then we went shopping to spend our $100 gift card!

Rentals

Renting a house or condo is another option. I've heard that VRBO (Vacation Rentals by Owner) is a great place to rent from but I've not used this site myself. Airbnb is another site to look in to.

Even though I know people who have good success with rental homes, I tend to shy away from renting houses from individuals because you never know if the house will smell like smoke, mold, pets, or air fresheners. All of the above would ruin it for me. However, ask around. You might find a house that someone else has stayed at with success, or you could question the owner about pets or fragrances used.

The positives are, when you stay at a house your kids can be as loud as they want! No need to worry about people in the next room or the people below you. And no loud noises waking you up throughout the night either.

We've rented a house through Eagle Ridge Resort in Galena, Illinois that is always nice because they run the vacation rental homes the same way they do the hotel rooms. So everything is nice and clean and maintained daily. If you're traveling with extended family, it's often cheaper to rent a house or villa and split the cost. Disney has a lot of villas as well. Just call Disney or call a Disney travel agent and inquire about the different options they have available in your price range.

Chapter 4
Accommodations without a Full Kitchen

If you have to stay in a regular hotel room, you can still eat clean. It just takes a little more effort. Call the hotel in advance and tell them you need a room with a mini refrigerator for medical reasons (your kids have food allergies or you need to keep medication refrigerated, etc.). If you tell them it is for medical reasons, they will usually supply you with a fridge at no extra charge.

Some hotels charge an extra $15 a day or so to have the fridge. This is when I'd make a note to myself, "Don't stay at this hotel again." It's best to find this information out at the time of booking. Also, I always call the day before we arrive to confirm the fridge will be in our room before we get there.

Having a microwave can be nice but we don't use a microwave for much. A lot of hotel rooms do have microwaves and fridges in every room but always ask when you book. Also ask if the fridge has a small freezer in it so you know for grocery shopping purposes. Most fridges have that tiny square freezer compartment, but not all.

This past summer, we stayed at Disney's Port Orleans Riverside Resort. It was a nice hotel but we had one issue. When we got to our room very late at night (about 10pm), I noticed that the fridge did not seem to have a freezer. We had just gone to Whole Foods and bought frozen berries for smoothies and a few other things that needed to go in a freezer.

23

I was told when I booked the room *and* when I called to confirm the day before, that it did have a freezer. It did not. They sent me a housekeeping employee who very rudely told me it did have a freezer. It did not but I was tired so I stuck my food in there and hoped for the best.

The next morning, our frozen berries were mush and the popsicles were liquid. Come to find out from management the next day, their fridges do *not* contain freezers anymore and the fridges only keep things moderately cold (interpret that: hardly cold at all). They do this to cut down on electrical costs. I had to put bags of ice over our turkey slices and change out the bag when the ice started to melt.

I had stuck a few things in a bucket of ice the night we arrived to try to keep them frozen so I brought those things to the front desk area where they have a hotel freezer. You can bring them your frozen items and they will give you a ticket. Then you have to go back and pick them up whenever you want them. So we did that. There's no charge for this service.

In the morning, I had to drive to the front reception building and get our frozen berries in order to make smoothies, and then drive the remainder back after making the smoothies. It was a pain but that's another option if you get stuck with a room without a freezer or fridge. You would need a car to make this feasible, although they do have buses that run back and forth to the front desk building but you may have to wait a little bit to catch one.

I went to the front desk and complained that I was not given the correct information at the time of booking so they refunded me the money I spent on my Whole Foods frozen items. They also refunded me the money we spent on breakfast at the Grand Floridian that first morning (about $75). The hotel itself was very nice and the kids and I loved it but the fridge experience didn't go over very well with this all natural mom.

If something is not up to your expectations at a Disney hotel, make sure to bring it up to the hotel manager because they will usually do what they can to make it right. They want to make sure their guests are happy. I just try to be nice about it.

Eating in Your Room

Eating out, especially at Disney, is very expensive so whatever you can bring or get on your own at the grocery store, is going to save you money. Breakfast is pretty easy. We'll sometimes do cereal, or oatmeal in the microwave. We like Gluten Freeda's apple cinnamon oatmeal packets. If your room doesn't have a microwave, sometimes you can get hot water or find a microwave at the hotel restaurant or food court.

This past year, I packed my Nutribullet blender in my suitcase. I like my smoothies. Or we'll do fresh fruit, muffins, Nature's Path Organic "Pop Tarts" or breakfast bars. You can also pick up some bagels at Einstein Bagels, Panera Bread, or Whole Foods. We get the blueberry, plain or cinnamon sugar bagels at Einstein Bagels. Not all of their bagels are free of the Big 3.

I also have a recipe for chocolate granola bars that my kids like. I'll usually pack a few of these from home in my backpack cooler.

For lunch and dinner, your options are a little more limited without a full kitchen. For lunch we usually do turkey slices, sandwiches, and fruit. If you're at the hotel for lunch, you can make Annie's microwavable mac-n-cheese. I pack a ceramic bowl and spoon for this and for the cereal. Microwave popcorn can be made for a snack.

If we're staying at a hotel room and we had to fly to get there, we just plan on eating out for lunch and dinner every day or you can order a pizza to the room. See chapter 5.

If you drive down to Disney, you could also bring along a crock pot or Instant Pot (my new love!). Don't forget to also bring down some of the ingredients you'll need like spices (preassembled ingredients are even better).

Most Disney hotels will have hot chocolate in the food court area so bring your own hot chocolate packets or homemade mix if your kids are going to want hot chocolate. You can get hot water in the food court. We picked up some Dandies marshmallows at Whole Foods.

Our hotel also did s'mores at night by a campfire so pick up some s'more ingredients if you plan on doing that, or bring some from home. We like Kinnikinnick's GFCF graham crackers, and you can use Enjoy Life chocolate chips or chocolate bars.

Disney Transportation

If you're staying at a Disney resort, you can use the Disney transportation system (buses) to get to and from all the Disney hotels and parks if you don't have a car. Just keep in mind that you will usually spend a little extra time on the buses than if you had your own car. Read more about the Disney transportation system and perks of staying at a Disney hotel in chapter 8.

Chapter 5

Eating Out

When vacationing, it's inevitable that you're probably going to eat out at some point, even if you have a full kitchen. Sometimes you don't have time to get back to your room and cook dinner, or sometimes you just don't want to! But try to plan eating out into your meal plan for the week. Below is a list of our favorite places to eat at in Orlando.

As I've stated, our family avoids the Big 3 (dyes, artificial flavors, and certain preservatives), and a few of us are also gluten and dairy free so these suggestions are based on what we can do and what we feel comfortable with. Just use common sense. If your child is gluten free, obviously you're going to avoid the bun if you're getting a hamburger. If you are a Feingold member, please refer to your Feingold Fast Food Shopping Guide for a full list of recommended fast foods.

Please research ingredients first on your own as ingredients can change at any time and each child can tolerate different amounts of cross contamination. If your child is very sensitive, avoid eating out completely as it is almost impossible to avoid cross contamination while eating out. We also typically avoid MSG and corn syrup but when eating out, these ingredients can sometimes be hard to avoid.

Chipotle

In 2015, Chipotle set off a chain reaction among restaurant chains by cleaning up their ingredients and removing GMO's (genetically modified ingredients) from their food. [1] Yay Chipotle!

Pretty much everything on Chipotle's menu is free of the Big 3. My kids and I get the chicken and rice burrito bowls. The chips and flour tortillas have recently undergone extensive revamping as of March, 2017. They have removed all preservatives. The flour tortillas now only contain five ingredients: wheat flour, water, non-GMO canola oil, and yeast.[2] We sometimes also do the chips and guacamole but there are a lot of cross-contamination issues with the chips if you are sensitive to gluten. If we're at home, we just order the guacamole and use Late July corn chips at home.

My kids like the Izze drinks here too. Blackberry Izze is my kids' favorite, or they have clean apple juice as well.

Cracker Barrel

I love Cracker Barrel! Some people do OK eating at Cracker Barrel and some don't. We do OK. They serve their pancakes with a mix of pure maple syrup and cane syrup. I buy their syrup to use at home sometimes. We usually get the pancakes or an omelet with sausage or bacon. Many people who avoid the Big 3 have done OK with their chicken and dumplings as well.

They have a lot of candy in their store that is free of the Big 3 as well. I like the Sunkist fruit gems and Clark candy bars (both contain corn syrup). My son likes the Valomilk chocolate marshmallow candy and the Snapple All Natural Jelly Bellies (check the label to make sure they are the natural ones that don't contain dyes). The last time we were there they also had some Black Forest organic gummy bears and gummy worms.

Five Guys Burgers and Fries

The bun may contain preservatives (Usually used in the pan spray when they bake them - they won't say.) but we are mostly gluten and dairy free anyway so we order just the patties and fries. You could bring your own bun if you wanted.

Their ketchup contains corn syrup so bring your own ketchup if you avoid corn syrup. Sometimes Whole Foods has corn syrup free ketchup packets at their restaurant and I'll grab a handful. Five Guys' fries are free of preservatives, which is rare. They cook the fries in peanut oil if you have a peanut allergy.

If you let your kids have pop, Coke and Sprite are free of the Big 3 but contain corn syrup. We just get water.

In-N-Out Burgers

We've not been here yet. They are more on the west coast in California but their burgers and fries are free of the Big 3 if you're heading to Disneyland in California.

McDonald's

Hamburgers at many fast food restaurants are free of the Big 3. We have done hamburgers at McDonald's, Wendy's, Burger King, and Culver's. Sometimes the pickles will have yellow dye but we order burgers plain or with ketchup only. The pickles at McDonald's and Wendy's do not contain yellow dye though.

Fries often contain BHT preservatives in the oil they are cooked in. McDonald's has a new campaign out saying they have removed the Big 3 from their chicken nuggets, hash browns, and fries and have also removed corn syrup from the hamburger buns. [3]

While this is a great move in the right direction, I'm still not willing to eat McDonald's regularly or the chicken nuggets at all due to other harmful ingredients still in these foods. My kids get a hamburger and apple juice and we skip the fries, and we only eat at McDonald's on very rare occasions.

Olive Garden

We do OK with Olive Garden's gluten free rotini with marinara sauce. I get gluten free grilled chicken added to mine. Many kids do fine with the regular noodles and either marina sauce or butter. Some people get fresh grated cheese on their pasta as well. The butter and cheese would be questionable but a lot of parents of kids who avoid the Big 3 have done OK with it. Most pasta in general is clean as pasta usually contains just a few basic ingredients.

You can also get plain chicken breasts seasoned with just salt and pepper, and steamed broccoli. The Olive Garden salad dressing contains corn syrup, dairy, and eggs and the natural flavors would be questionable so that's at your own discretion.

My son does eat the breadsticks but I don't know for sure if they are clean or not. I figure, we're on vacation and we're not going to be eating perfectly the entire time. We make sure to take digestive enzymes when eating out though (see chapter 9).

Panera Bread

In 2016, Panera Bread cleaned up their menu, removing the Big 3 from many of their items.[4] The one thing they do not mention is the removal of TBHQ. This can be used in the frying oil or pan oil but it seems most of their items are pretty clean so I feel safe eating most items off their menu.

My son likes their chicken noodle soup and Turkey Bacon Bravo sandwiches, and I get their BBQ chicken salad (has dairy) or their Strawberry Poppy Seed Chicken salad in the summer. Many kids do well with their macaroni and cheese and they have a lot of baked goods that are clean as well. We've only done the bagels from the bakery but the cookies and brownies appear to be clean.

Papa John's Pizza

Papa John's used to be Feingold acceptable for years when we first started the Feingold Diet in 2005, and then suddenly they disappeared from the Feingold Fast Food Shopping Guide. I contacted Papa John's directly and they claimed they are free of the

Big 3 including the pan sprays they use. They actually said they do not use pans at all. [5]

In 2016, Papa John's removed 14 unhealthy ingredients but we still stick to the cheese pizzas only. [6] You can check out the list of ingredients on their web site to see what your family can do. You can have Papa John's delivered to your hotel room. They have many locations in Orlando

We get the hand-tossed cheese pizzas and request pizza sauce on the side instead of garlic sauce. The garlic sauce used to contain dyes but they have since removed the dyes from the garlic sauce. The garlic sauce contains natural flavors though which could be questionable. [7] When we avoided salicylates, we would order a cheese pizza with no sauce, extra cheese, and then I would make a garlic butter dipping sauce (recipe in my first book, "All Natural Mom's Guide to the Feingold Diet."). I told my son it was like garlic bread with cheese.

Starbuck's

I don't drink coffee so we never go to Starbuck's but they have a lot of breakfast items, sandwiches, and baked goods that are free of the Big 3 (some have corn syrup). If you are a Feingold member, check out your Fast Food Guide. Sometimes near the check out, they have Justin's peanut butter cups.

If I were to take my son there, I think he would try the following: Slow Roasted Ham and Swiss breakfast sandwich, blueberry muffin, Chocolate Croissant (has corn syrup), blueberry scone, plain bagel, Old-Fashioned Grilled Cheese, BBQ Beef Brisket on Sourdough, or a Ham and Swiss Panini (corn syrup). [8]

For dessert, he'd probably try the Classic Coffeecake, Old-Fashioned Glazed Doughnut (corn syrup), Double Chocolate Brownie, Gluten-Free Marshmallow Dream Bar (corn syrup), Salted Caramel Square with Pecans (corn syrup), or a Chocolate Chip Cookie or Frosted Snowman Cookie (both have corn syrup).[8]

Starbuck's has their menu and ingredients posted on their web site under "Menu." I would go online and look at the ingredients they have posted to see what your family can eat or drink there.

Subway

Not much here is gluten and dairy free but my oldest does some of their sandwiches. He gets the Italian bread as it does not contain corn syrup. Their cheese pizza is also currently free of the Big 3 and they have Lay's potato chips and a few clean juices.

If you are a Feingold member, check your Fast Food Guide as there are random things that Feingold recommends from here. Many of the deli meats currently contain preservatives. I get the meatball sandwich sometimes. My son used to get the grilled chicken strips on Italian bread.

Subway has announced that they will be removing artificial colors, flavors, and preservatives from their food by 2017 so watch for that.[9] I'm always skeptical at first because what a big company like Subway considers preservatives and what I consider harmful preservatives could differ, but I'm excited that more companies are making these changes.

Taco Bell and Pizza Hut are two other companies who have made similar claims to clean up their ingredients in the near future.

Wendy's

Wendy's claims to have removed the preservative TBHQ from their "natural cut" fries but some local restaurants are still using cooking oil that contains TBHQ so question the manager first. [10] The remaining ingredients are not healthy so we just skip the fries.

We usually get a double stack without cheese or a bun, or a regular hamburger. The Homestyle Spicy Chicken sandwich and Spicy Chicken Nuggets are also free of the Big 3. Baked potatoes are another option, as well as salad. I like Ranch dressing (has MSG), or they have Lemon Garlic Caesar (has corn syrup), or Pomegranate Vinaigrette that are also free of the Big 3.

Disney Resort Restaurants

For most Disney hotel restaurants, you'll want to make reservations ahead of time, especially for any Disney character restaurants. Some of them fill up as quickly as six months in advance. Disney is very accommodating for food allergies. Just ask for their allergy menu or ask to talk to the chef. You may want to call ahead and talk to them as well so you know what you can expect. If you've made a reservation in advance, send an e-mail to specialdiets@disneyworld.com at least 14 days prior to your reservation to go over your order and allergies. For more on eating at Disney, see chapter 6.

Bringing along an "Avoid the Big 3" magnet (shown below) can be helpful to let the chef know what you avoid. If you don't avoid salicylates, just tell them to ignore the right side of the magnet or put a post-it note over that half with a big "X" just to avoid any confusion. You can purchase these magnets on my web site.

Avoid "The Big 3"	List of Common Salicylates
1. All Dyes Such as Red #40, Yellow FD&C #6, Blue #1, Tartrazine, "Colors Added" Caramel Color (questionable) **2. Artificial Flavors** Vanillin Artificial flavors or "flavors added" Natural flavors (sometimes questionable but more often OK) **3. Preservatives** BHT, BHA, and TBHQ (sometimes not listed)	**LOW** Pears, lemons, limes, watermelon, honeydew, pomegranate, mango, kiwi, papaya, asparagus, Brussel sprouts, broccoli, cauliflower, green beans, kale, lettuce, onions, peas, sweet potato, carrots, pumpkin, cashews, pecans, sunflower seeds **MEDIUM** Bananas, cantaloupe, avocado, canned pineapple, grapefruit, white potatoes, spinach, honey **HIGH** Apples, grapes, raisins, all berries, cherries, apricots, oranges, peaches, plums, prunes, dates, fresh pineapple, cucumbers, pickles, peppers, tomatoes, zucchini, almonds, molasses, clover honey, tea, coffee

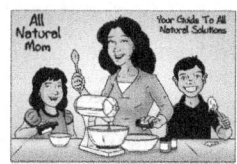

To learn more about the Feingold Diet,
visit my blog at www.allnaturalmomof4.com

The biggest drawback to eating at Disney is they are very expensive. I think we'd also get tired of eating at Disney restaurants every day because their selection of allergy-friendly food isn't huge. It's also not the best food I've ever tasted either. One or two meals is fine, but personally, if I had to eat at a Disney restaurant for every meal, every day, I think I'd get sick of it so we opted not to do their meal plan packages. Some families have done the meal packages though and have been happy with their experience, so it's a personal decision.

My kids usually get the hamburgers with gluten free buns and gluten free fries. Some people will do plain grilled chicken, plain baked potatoes, noodles with butter, steak, or fish, just depending on what your kids like. But, talk to the chef and see what they can come up with.

Breakfast at Disney Resorts

We have done the character breakfasts and you can expect Mickey pancakes or waffles. They can make the pancakes and waffles gluten and dairy free. They use a GFCF Namaste pancake mix which is what I use at home. They also usually have cinnamon sugar Kinnikinnick doughnuts which are free of the Big 3 and gluten and dairy free.

We've done Denver omelets, hash brown potatoes and fresh fruit. They told us they use Earth Balance soy and dairy free butter for the hash browns. Just make sure when you order to tell them what ingredients you avoid and make sure to ask for pure maple syrup as the regular syrup will have artificial flavor and lots of corn syrup.

Last summer we ate breakfast at the Grand Floridian Café and it was good. We ordered off the menu. For the four of us, it was about $75. After breakfast my daughter wanted to play in the sand on their beach. Warning: Don't go near the water! A few days after we were there, we heard on the news that a little boy was snatched and killed by an alligator as he was wading in the water on that same beach. So sad!

They've since put up warning signs and blocked off some areas, but being from Chicago and not being familiar with alligators, I would've let my daughter wade in the water too if she wanted. Thank goodness she didn't want to! She has a fear of sharks and open water!

Dessert at Disney Resorts

You can almost always find some Enjoy Life cookies around Disney. One year at the Disney Caribbean Beach Resort food court, we found some brownies. They were the prepackaged French Meadow brand, which are GFCF and free of the Big 3.

However, it seems they've replaced the French Meadow brand with OMG brand brownies and chocolate chip cookies. These are gluten free but not dairy free. We choose to stay away from the OMG brand desserts because they contain dairy and also natural flavors (which can be questionable), but take a look at the ingredients to see if it's something your kids can do.

Some Disney sit down restaurants will have Namaste chocolate cake which is gluten and dairy free and free of the Big 3. They'll usually also have Rice Dream dairy free vanilla ice cream. Just ask your server about it.

If your kids can do dairy, I would head over to Disney Springs to Haagen-Dazs for ice cream and skip dessert at the Disney resort restaurants. (See next section.)

Disney Springs (formerly known as Downtown Disney)

When we go to the Disney Springs shopping area, there are a few places that we always stop.

Wetzel's Pretzels

They have a stand that sells fresh lemonade. Just double check and make sure they are still only using fresh lemons, water, and sugar. They had Dragonfruit Glaceau Vitamin water here as well. Make sure you get the regular and not the Zero version if they have both.

Erin McKenna's Bakery

This used to be Babycakes Bakery. They have a very tiny "Bakery" sign on a brick building that is easy to miss but it's across from a restaurant called The Boathouse and near Paddlefish (formerly named Fulton's Crab House.) Paddlefish can be more easily seen when you are walking through Disney Springs.

This bakery sells gluten and dairy free donuts, cupcakes, and other baked goods that are also free of the Big 3. If you have a child with food allergies, this a definite must-stop location. My daughter likes the mint frosted chocolate cupcakes. Sometimes they have chocolate brownie cupcakes. These are good but super sweet. My kids like the regular chocolate cupcakes with chocolate frosting the best but sometimes they have limited availability.

We've tried the donuts. We don't care for the chocolate frosted ones but I like the vanilla or raspberry frosted ones. Then we go to Wetzel's Pretzels and get lemonade!

Check out their web site at www.erinmckennasbakery.com/orlando/ to check out some of their treats and list of ingredients before heading there. They also sell some of their bakery items like their mini brownie cupcakes at various Disney locations such as Disney's Beach Resort and Disney's Boardwalk Bakery.

Ghirardelli's

Some of Ghirardelli's chocolates are free of the Big 3. You'll have to read the labels and look out for vanillin and TBHQ but some of the more plain varieties of wrapped chocolates are clean. Ghirardelli's is located near the World of Disney and close to the stage where they have performances.

Haagen-Dazs Ice Cream

There is a Haagen Dazs ice cream shop on the west side of Disney Springs. (They call it Disney Springs West Side.) Several flavors of their ice cream are free of the Big 3 but some contain corn syrup. I never had my Feingold book on me so we always just stuck to either vanilla or chocolate ice cream because my son was happy with that and I knew those flavors didn't have corn syrup.

But other options currently free of the Big 3 are butter pecan, cookies and cream, peanut butter pie, and deep chocolate peanut butter, to name a few. If you are a Feingold member, check your Foodlist and Shopping Guide for more options.

Haagen-Dazs ice cream bars are also free of the Big 3 if you happen to find those anywhere else. Many grocery stores carry them.

World of Disney

At the World of Disney (a store at Disney Springs) we found some dye-free lollipops. I think this was the highlight of the entire trip for my kids! More info on the dye free lollipops in chapter 6.

Random Tip: Not Disney-related, but if you happen to be going to Universal Studios or Islands of Adventure theme parks as well, they have frozen Cokes that my kids have done well with.

Chapter 6
Eating at the Parks

If you have a full kitchen, you can bring your lunch and dinner with you to the parks. Disney lets you bring food in at Magic Kingdom. They just don't allow glass items or the hard plastic coolers. Make sure your cooler is small enough to fit in one of their lockers if you need to store it in a locker. We use a backpack cooler.

We've always had a stroller with us so we haven't used the lockers yet. The nice part of having a stroller is you can carry all your food and drinks around with you all day. No need to run back to the lockers. If you didn't bring a stroller down with you, you can rent a stroller from the park, but they're expensive.

For any other parks that don't allow food in, just tell the security person that your kids have food allergies and medically necessary diets. Sometimes this is all you need to do and they'll let you through. We've never had a problem once.

Remember, due to HIPAA laws, they aren't allowed to question what medical condition your child has. Keep in mind though that some theme parks such as Six Flags Great America are now requiring a doctor's note that simply says that your child has a condition (do not name the condition) that requires them to bring their own food. As of 2017, Disney does *not* require a doctor's note.[1]

What to Pack

I always pack insulated food thermoses from home for the parks. I've filled thermoses with spaghetti, chili, mac-n-cheese, chicken and rice, hot dogs (I fill the thermos with hot water to keep the hot dogs hot), soup, etc. I like the thermoses that I get online. The character ones at Target are small and don't keep the food as warm, or warm for as long.

We usually pack sandwiches too, and lots of cut up fruit. I use Tupperware containers so the sandwiches and fruit don't get smashed in the cooler. And we bring lots of snacks too and usually a can of pop from Whole Foods as a treat for the kids to share.

We usually end up bringing our lunch and eating dinner at the park but we've packed both lunch and dinner before as well. That was easier when I only had one or two kids to feed! If you don't have a full kitchen, you can pick up some things at Whole Foods to bring with or make sandwiches.

Eating at the Park Restaurants

In 2015, Disney launched its allergy-friendly menus. At each restaurant, when you go to order, they will call out an allergy chef or special-diet trained cast member to go over the allergy-friendly menu with you and take your order. Be aware that your allergy-friendly meal may take longer than the rest of your family's order.

If you only avoid gluten, dairy, or eggs, you can easily see from the menu what your child can or can't eat. If you also avoid the Big 3 though, you will have slightly fewer options and will have to question Disney a little more on the ingredients.

Below are some of the places we've eaten at inside Magic Kingdom but you'll find similar options at the other Disney parks. Disney changes things up a bit from time to time but as of 2017, this is what is being served where. Check out the web sites I have listed in chapter 10 for information on specific food allergens and to view menus at the restaurants you plan on going to.

And again, if you are eating out, you are taking a risk. It's best to bring your own food, but when you need to eat at the parks, below are some options that many kids who avoid the Big 3, including my own, have typically had success with.

Galactic Grill

Galactic Grill is located in Tomorrowland near the Toy Story attraction. We usually bring our lunch and then do gluten free hamburgers here for dinner. They currently use EnerG gluten free buns. The burgers come with gluten free fries, and grapes. Make sure to specify if you have gluten and dairy allergies. [2]

The fries are questionable as they could be cooked in oil which contains TBHQ or another preservative but we take the risk. They also have GFCF chocolate chip cookies and OMG brownies. As I mentioned in chapter 5, the gluten free OMG brownies contain dairy and natural flavors which would be questionable.

They also offer a chopped salad with grilled chicken that is gluten and dairy free. I would bring my own salad dressing though.

Cosmic Ray's

Also located in Tomorrowland near Space Mountain, this restaurant also serves gluten free hamburgers and fries, and a GFCF chocolate chip cookie. [3]

Jumbo Turkey Legs

My kids love these. I think they just like the novelty of eating a gigantic "chicken" leg. These are gluten and dairy free and likely free of the Big 3. You can find them at a food cart in Frontierland. [4]

Cinderella's Royal Table

Magic Kingdom also has character dining but you usually need to book it months in advance (you can request reservations up to 180 days in advance). They are open for breakfast, lunch, and dinner. Cinderella's Royal Table is located inside Cinderella's castle. We had dinner here when my daughter was 4. She loved it. We got to take pictures with Cinderella, and some of the Cinderella characters came out briefly during dinner.

The chefs can customize your meal to your specifications in the back. For lunch and dinner they typically serve things like fish, chicken, steak, roast beef, turkey, mashed potatoes, spaghetti, and/or allergy-friendly chicken tenders (see Liberty Tree Tavern section). [5]

The menu changes periodically so call ahead and talk to a special diet cast member who can send you the current allergy-friendly menu and go over your options. They can cut your meat in the back to avoid some of the seasonings in the gravies and sauces that may contain chemicals or gluten and dairy.

For dessert, most restaurants will have Enjoy Life cookies on hand. They can make an ice cream cookie sandwich out of two chocolate chip or sugar cookies and some vanilla Rice Dream dairy free ice cream.

One family had the chef make their child chocolate mousse with fresh raspberries (free of the big 3 but not dairy free). They also have some GFCF mini chocolate cakes made from a Namaste cake mix. [5]

Liberty Tree Tavern

You usually need a reservation here as well but we've walked in before. This is a nicer sit down restaurant where you have a waiter or waitress. They serve things like prime rib, pork roast, turkey, grilled chicken, mashed potatoes, green beans, gluten free chicken tenders, or a gluten free chicken patty on a gluten free bun. [6]

The chicken tenders are Allergy Free Foods brand and are GFCF but "may" contain some chemicals in the seasonings but I'd consider it to be a better option than most of the regular park food. We have not tried the chicken tenders yet. My kids usually get the roasted turkey or prime rib, mashed potatoes (make sure to tell them if you are dairy free), and green beans.

Tony's Town Square Restaurant

This is an Italian restaurant near the entrance to Magic Kingdom. Advanced reservations recommended here as well. They serve gluten free (and regular) spaghetti and meatballs here. They use Tinkyada brown rice noodles for the gluten free pasta. They also serve steak and fish here. If you happen to be eating while the parade is going on, ask to sit near the window. [7]

Peco's Bill Tall Tale Inn & Cafe

Peco's Bill serves Tex-Mex cuisine and is located in Frontierland. We have not eaten at this restaurant but we may try it next time. I have one child who is obsessed with just plain white rice. If you are gluten, dairy and egg free, they have a chicken, beef, or vegetarian white rice bowl. The regular seasoned rice contains dairy. They also have some sides that may be OK like black beans and guacamole. [8]

I would have to question how they season their meat though before we tried it. It may contain preservatives and artificial flavors but it's possible they don't. They also have Enjoy Life GFCF chocolate chip cookies here and Simply brand orange juice which my kids love.

Treats at the Parks

What kid doesn't love treats? And it's always even more exciting for allergy kids when they can find something in a store that they can actually have. Below are some of the treats we've found around the parks.

Walker's Shortbread Cookies

Our first stop at Magic Kingdom is always the confectionary store near the entrance. Here they have Mickey Walker shortbread round cookies. They contain just flour, sugar, salt, and butter. [9] My son used to love getting these when he was little.

Dye Free Lollipops

Last year, Disney came out with dye and artificial flavor free lollipops! They're the big round swirl suckers. We found them at the Disney parks, at Disney Springs (World of Disney shop), and at a shop on Disney's Boardwalk.

They have strawberry and lemon flavors. They do contain corn syrup and one of the ingredients is natural flavors which could potentially have an artificial flavor in it but I'm going to guess (and hope) that it doesn't. Just make sure to read the labels as they sell both the dye-free and the regular suckers as well.

A few chemical-sensitive families have tried the new suckers and their kids did OK with them. I had another allergy mom mail me some for Christmas. My kids loved them! And no big reactions.

This year my daughter also found a candy tube with a fan on the end that had small round candies inside that were dye-free. The ingredients read clean with natural flavors being the only questionable ingredient so we tried them out and did OK with them. We found it at World of Disney at Disney Springs. Glad to see Disney jumping on the dye-free bandwagon!

Frozen Strawberry Fruit Bars

This year, I stopped by an ice cream cart in Disney Springs and asked to see the ingredients on their frozen strawberry fruit bars. Sometimes they are all natural and sometimes they are not. This time we got lucky and it was all natural and no corn syrup. The brand was Helados Mexico. I have checked these ice cream carts at Magic Kingdom before and it's always hit or miss. I look for one that has cane sugar instead of corn syrup, no red dyes or artificial flavors, and no artificial sweeteners like aspartame or sucralose.

Bring Your Own

You can also bring along some of your own treats too. They sell Mickey shaped rice krispy treats. Next time we go, I plan to make my own at home. I have a Mickey shaped sandwich bread cutter that I use to cut out rice krispy treats in the shape of Mickey just like they sell in the store.

Wrap it in Saran Wrap, stick a Mickey sticker on it and call it a day! Depending on your kids' ages, they'll never know the difference. Just keep in mind that homemade rice krispy treats get stale within a day or two so you may have to make them in Florida.

Or make some Mickey shaped sugar cookies at home and bring them with. Just don't show your kids until you get to the parks. Yum Earth suckers, Surf Sweet gummy worms, Lovely fruit chews, and K-Too "Oreos" are some other treats that we might bring along as well. And then as I've mentioned, they have Enjoy Life cookies (which are GFCF and free of the Big 3) at various places throughout Disney, and vanilla Rice Dream ice cream at several of the restaurants.

48

Chapter 7
Disney Cruising

In March, 2012 we went on a 3-night cruise on the Disney Dream out of Florida, which was one of the larger, newer ships. My kids were 15 months, 5, 8, and 11 at the time. It was a little hectic for me but the kids enjoyed it. I would not take a toddler on a cruise again but it was gifted to us so it was hard to refuse.

I prefer a regular cruise over Disney as Disney charges much more than other cruise lines. I don't feel the increased cost is justified, especially considering Disney's food is not great in my opinion, but we did have a good time.

We just did another 3-night Disney cruise in March, 2017 and this time we were on the Disney Wonder which is a smaller ship so it had fewer passengers sharing a similar sized pool and pool chairs. We didn't have a hard time at all finding space in the pool or empty pool chairs. The waterslide on the Wonder is not as glamorous but my kids only waited a few minutes to go down it as opposed to the hour wait on the Disney Dream for the Aquaduck waterslide.

This last cruise, my youngest was 6. It was much more fun for me this time as I didn't have to go back to the room for my daughter's naps and early bed time. The night time entertainment begins around 8:30pm and lasts till midnight so traveling with little ones can make it difficult to enjoy all the offerings on a cruise unless you have grandparents or a babysitter along.

I recommend requesting the early dinner seating which is around 6:00pm. There is a nightly show for the 6:00pm dinner seating around 8:30pm every night which gives you just enough time to go back to your room and change after dinner if you want. The ship can get cold sometimes later at night. The later dinner seating is around 8:00pm.

The Food

I'm sorry to say, but I can't boast about Disney's food. In my opinion, it's average at best, when dealing with food allergies at least. I've cruised with Royal Caribbean and Carnival and I think they do a better job as far as food quality.

I'll first cover cruising when on a gluten and dairy free diet as that is what we have the most experience with. If you are just avoiding the Big 3 (dyes, artificial flavors, and preservatives), you will have a few more options.

Keep in mind, when you cruise, you are at the mercy of those preparing your food. You don't get the chance to go back in the kitchen and look at all the list of ingredients. But, if you let your waiter know what you avoid, they do their best to avoid those ingredients.

On Disney, each night for dinner you will dine in a different dining room with a different chef but with the same waiter. We ended up eating some of the same foods over and over because their selection of gluten and dairy free food is limited.

So for dinner, it was lots of steak, plain chicken breasts, gluten free spaghetti, and plain baked potatoes. My kids tried the hamburgers on gluten free buns one night and they were awful. The meat was like a McDonald's hamburger and the bun was super hard. They should have used an Udi's bun and heated it up. If your kids like fish (mine don't), that's another good option.

We tried out the gluten free dinner rolls the first night and told them to keep them the next night. They were dry and tasteless, and they didn't even bother to heat them up. They tasted like hamburger buns, which is what they should have used on the hamburgers. I couldn't wait to get home and eat some good food with some flavor! My kids did not enjoy the food on the cruise either. They must be spoiled with good cooking at home!

Gluten and dairy free doesn't have to be plain and boring. For a company as large as Disney, I was disappointed that they didn't have chefs that could do more with a GFCF diet. I wanted to get in that kitchen and give them some of my recipes! We couldn't possibly be the only guests with gluten and dairy allergies.

Dessert

Dessert was always the same thing - Namaste GFCF chocolate cake and Rice Dream dairy free vanilla ice cream. The last night my kids couldn't stand the thought of more chocolate cake so I asked if they had any GFCF cookies. I knew Disney usually had Enjoy Life cookies at the parks. So our waiter brought us out a plate of Enjoy Life Snickerdoodle cookies. Nothing special but my kids ate them. It was better than the same old chocolate cake again.

If I could offer some dessert suggestions to Disney, here's what I would suggest: Chocolate covered strawberries using Enjoy Life dairy free chocolate chips, or heat up some Immaculate GFCF chocolate chip cookies, or put together a cute display of cut up fruit with a fruity dressing and some Soyatoo dairy free whip cream, or So Delicious ice cream bars to substitute the Mickey ice cream bars the other kids on the ship get.

And, I would kindly let them know there are other flavors of dairy free ice cream besides vanilla! There's So Delicious Salted Caramel Cluster or Luna and Larry's Dark Chocolate Coconut Bliss ice cream. I digress. But if they can make a Namaste cake mix, they can certainly make other things.

I can't imagine if we went on a 7-day cruise. I would be so sick of the monotony of food choices. They need to hire me as a special diet consultant to their chefs! I'll work for free. Scratch that. I'll work for free Disney cruises for life! Hold the Namaste chocolate cake. (For the record, we actually like the Namaste chocolate cake, but after eating it three days in a row, it grows tiresome!)

I think it was also harder on my kids because of the fact that we had other relatives at our table who were not gluten and dairy free and they saw all the different variety of desserts they were getting - ice cream sundaes with whip cream and cookies, strawberry shortcake, apple pie, tiramisu, etc.

Disney does aim to please so if we ever do a Disney cruise again, I'd consider sending a list of recommendations and recipes ahead of time.

And, like almost all cruises, Disney has a self-serve soft serve ice cream station near the pools. This of course would not be free of the Big 3.

My kids are used to not having ice cream so it didn't bother them but they do also have a place that makes smoothies near the pool. The crew members can make them dairy free as well. This is a nice alternative to ice cream as you can tell them what to put in your smoothie.

Breakfast

I think next time we would try to do breakfast on our own in our rooms for the kids instead of at the buffet every day. Or even preorder room service (room service takes a long time to get to your room FYI). The breakfast buffet had Krispy Kreme style doughnuts every day, pancakes, and eggs, etc. I think it was hard for my kids to see and walk past the doughnuts. I know it was hard for me!

You can preorder GFCF waffles or pancakes at your dinner the night before. They use a Namaste pancake mix. We had them add some dairy free chocolate chips as well. Or you can have them add fresh blueberries or strawberries. The kids liked the waffles but didn't want them every day. Expect to wait a few minutes for them to bring you the special pre-orders though. The first day we had to wait 10 minutes because we didn't pre-order them. The next day it was only a few minutes.

When you arrive at the buffet, you just notify one of the kitchen staff that you made a pre-order (tell them your waiter's name) and they'll call down to the dining room and have your order brought up.

It was hard for my kids to wait for their waffles while everyone else in our party was busy eating already. One day they also brought my kids some GFCF cinnamon doughnuts heated up while we were waiting. We have these at home so they weren't too much of a novelty to my kids.

The buffet also had fresh fruit and potatoes. I'm not sure if the potatoes at the buffet were GFCF (they may have been cooked in butter), but that's something you could probably preorder GFCF as well if you'd like.

You also have the option of eating in the dining room for breakfast with a waiter, but we were never up in time to make it to the dining room. The buffet was open till 10:45am every morning.

Lunch on the Private Island

Disney has a private island in Cococay, Bahamas. They serve you lunch on the island, buffet style. They had BBQ ribs (not sure if these were free of the Big 3. I would ask to see the ingredients on the BBQ sauce.), corn on the cob (may have dairy), hamburgers, rice, fish, chili, and other sides. We did the hamburgers and corn. If you want gluten free hamburger buns, you will have to pre-order that the night before with your waiter.

For dessert, we pre-ordered Namaste chocolate cake and Rice Dream ice cream. You just have to find your waiter out there or let another Disney cast member know. The ice cream was pretty well melted as they have to bring it from the ship. They also bring out the soft serve ice cream stations FYI. Next time, I think I'll bring out a treat of our own for my kids like K-Too "Oreos" or candy.

FYI - if you buy anything on the private island, make sure you pay cash! We charged something small to our room from a little shop that totaled around $14 and they added another $26 in Bahamian island tax! Something we would have noticed had we paid cash. This was not a Disney owned shop. You could tell it was a shop owned by a local.

My girls also got their hair braided here. I would not do braiding in Nassau, Bahamas, which is the first stop on the 3-day cruises out of Florida. I don't trust that their combs are totally sanitary.

Notifying Disney of Food Allergies

Many people ask if we had to notify Disney in advance of our food allergies. For our first cruise, I did when I booked the room. It was listed on our reservation and the waiters had us marked as gluten and dairy free. They take this very seriously we found out!

About half way through our first cruise, I decided I couldn't take the GFCF food they were feeding me anymore, and I'd rather just eat the regular gluten and dairy filled food because I was starving, and I was on a cruise with all you can eat food! So I asked for one of the other things on the menu for that night. They refused! And the waiter argued with me.

He said when I booked the room, I stated I was GFCF and they could not serve me anything but GFCF food. He could lose his job. Ugh! At that moment, I knew exactly how my kids felt! I wanted to eat what everyone else was having! With my kids, I try to make sure that whatever they are having is better than what everyone else is having though. This trip, I could not.

For our second cruise, I did not tell them ahead of time that we were GFCF. I just talked to our waiter the first night. Next time, I will talk to the waiter prior to dinner so they can prepare some things ahead of time. Certain things like the gluten free spaghetti and GFCF chocolate cake needed to be pre-ordered the night before.

Each night I would look at the menu for the following night and see if we could eat anything on the menu or if we wanted to special order anything. My younger daughter didn't like anything but the spaghetti. The spaghetti sauce was not very good but my daughter ate it.

One night I just let the kids get regular macaroni and cheese because they didn't want anything else (and I couldn't blame them). We took some Houston AFP Peptizyde digestive enzymes.

Hindsight, I would have supplemented more with our own snacks and treats. They had a mini fridge in the room. Our first cruise, I didn't think we could bring food on board and I was just hoping they'd be able to figure out what to feed us.

For our second cruise, I did bring some food, but you are supposed to only bring prepackaged foods, not homemade. They didn't say anything at security though and nothing was manually searched. All of our belongings just went through a security scanner. We also brought along a case of water bottles.

If You Do Not Have Food Allergies

If you do not have food allergies but just avoid the Big 3, just talk to your waiter and let them know what you avoid and what kinds of foods your kids like. They should be able to come up with some ideas of what your kids can eat fairly easily. Desserts are a little more of a challenge but it can be done. Sometimes they'll make a pudding or chocolate mousse from scratch or do something with fruit. Or, bring along some of your own desserts.

Movies and Popcorn

Disney has a nice movie theater where they show Disney movies. We got to see the new Beauty and the Beast movie just after it came out. Right outside the theater, they give out popcorn which likely contains dyes and artificial flavors. So, just be aware of this and bring your own popcorn or snacks if you'd like.

Meet and Greets

On our first cruise, we were disappointed with the meet and greets for the Disney characters. I had this idea that characters would be walking around the ship all the time. That was not the case.

They had set times when you could meet the characters and take pictures with them. They seemed to always be at inconvenient times (like when the ship was docked at the private island). When we could make it, there were long lines and sometimes the line would abruptly shut down before we got up to the character. My daughter was disappointed.

Our second cruise, our travel agent, Larissa Boland told me we could make reservations for the meet and greets. Yay. I totally forgot about it though. But it worked out because we happened to be on our way out to the island and saw the Disney princesses before leaving the ship, so we got in line (and the line was short because most people were already out on the island. We're late risers.). The guy asked if we had reservations and I said I did but left our tickets in the room. He said that was fine because he had plenty of room for walk-ups.

But, all in all, we had a good time. In my experience, I would say that it's difficult to stay on a special diet on a cruise 100% of the time due to the fact that you have such little control over the food situation. But, I do know many families who have done so and have had a very good experience, so it's definitely possible. If you have a Disney cruise planned, I hope some of these tips will be helpful.

Chapter 8
Tips for Disney

Disney changes policies quickly so please double check and confirm all info before your trip. See chapter 10 for a list of good resources for vacation planning purposes.

Best Time of Year to Visit Disney

There are certainly better times of the year to visit Disney than others. In general, if kids are out of school, like for summer break (mid-June to mid-August are the busiest times), spring break, Thanksgiving break, or Christmas break, the parks are going to be extremely crowded. We avoid going to the parks during these times (because we've done it before and spent most of our day standing in lines). Disney also takes the liberty of raising their ticket prices during peak seasons.

We also try to visit the parks midweek like Tuesday, Wednesday, or Thursday, as opposed to the weekend or a Monday or Friday when the parks are usually busier. [1]

You'll also want to check Disney's calendar of events as well for the week you plan on going. Sometimes they have big events going on which could affect crowd sizes at the parks. I know Disney Gay Days in Orlando is the first week of June. [2] Gay Days in California is the beginning of October. This is not a Disney-sponsored event but it is an organized event that can draw a big crowd.

Summers in Florida also get very hot. We avoid going past mid-June. If you do go in the summer, save yourself some money and sanity by buying a water bottle with a fan on it before you go, and make sure you remember to bring it with you to the parks.

Halloween at Disney

My favorite time of year to go is in the fall or in May. We went over Halloween one year as my kids were off school for two days for parent teacher conferences. I made my 4-year old daughter at the time, an appointment with Bibbidi Bobbidi Boutique (6 months in advance!) in Disney Springs and she dressed up as Cinderella for Halloween.

We went trick-or-treating in Celebration (a community of homes built by Disney). And no, my kids don't eat most of the candy, but they have fun collecting it. For tips on how to do Halloween on a special diet or when you are dye-free, check out my next book, *"Living Dye-Free in a Cotton Candy World"* coming in 2017.

They also had trick-or-treating at the Disney parks all week. They call it, "Mickey's Not So Scary Halloween Party" which begins the end of August and runs through November 1st. They offer some allergy-friendly treats now as well, which is new and very cool! [3]

Your child will get a teal treat bag so that cast members will know to give your child a teal token instead of candy. At the end of the day, your child can take those tokens and exchange them for candy at a designated location. The options in 2016 were Surf Sweet gummy worms, gummy bears, or jelly beans, Enjoy Life dairy free chocolate bars, Enjoy Life cookies, Smarties, or a craft kit. Obviously we'd pass on the dye-filled Smarties. [3]

Fast Passes

If you've not been to Disney for a while, they have implemented a newer Fast Pass system. Each ticket holder is allowed three free fast passes which allows them to get on rides without much wait using the Fast Pass lanes. You have to reserve these though ahead of time.

If you are staying at a Disney hotel, you can reserve your fast pass rides and times starting 60 days in advance. If you are not staying at a Disney hotel, or you have a season pass, you can reserve your fast passes up to 30 days in advance. Some of the more popular rides fill up quick so make sure you book yours as soon as you're able to. [4]

After you use up your three fast passes, you're allowed to book more fast passes, one at a time using the kiosks at the parks (which sometimes have long lines and a lot of times all of the rides are already gone), or using a Disney app. So, keep that in mind when you are booking your initial three fast passes. If you book the last one for 8:00pm, you won't be able to try to get another fast pass until after that last one is used. If you book all three fast passes before 1:00pm, then you can try to get more after your last ride at 1:00pm.

Disability Pass

If you have a child with a disability such as autism, you can request a disability pass at Guest Services when you get to the parks. Kids with autism, Lyme, or PANDAS (Pediatric Autoimmune Neurological Disorder Associated With Strep) often have a hard time waiting in lines and can get overstimulated easily from all the commotion that is Disney. [5]

Without the disability pass, lasting a whole day at Disney may not happen and you pay a lot of money for your tickets. My daughter also has hypotonia which is low muscle tone, making it hard for her to walk for long periods of time. When she was little, we just had her sit in the stroller, but as she got older and bigger that was no longer an option, and she didn't want to use a wheelchair.

As of 2017, a doctor's note is not required at Disney for a disability pass. They may ask the nature of the disability. They are just asking so they know what kind of disability pass to give you. For example, if your child needs a wheelchair or needs to use their stroller as a wheelchair, they will give you a special tag for that as well. [5]

Right now, Disney offers all ticket holders three free fast passes. The disability pass works somewhat similar to the fast pass. [5] You can only use one at a time. You walk up to the ride you want to go on and show them your disability pass. They will write down a return time (usually with an hour window). This time usually correlates with the actual wait time. So if the wait time is 30 minutes and it is noon, they'll tell you to come back between 12:30pm and 1:30pm. While we were waiting, we would use one of our regular fast passes. This worked well. We seemed to go straight from our disability pass ride to our fast pass ride without much waiting in between.

Souvenir Pickup

Here's something I didn't know! Merchandise purchased throughout the day can be delivered up to the front of the park at a designated location, to be picked up on your way out of the park. Just let your retail clerk know at the time of purchase. I would have taken advantage of this service as we tend to buy a lot of souvenirs as a substitute to buying treats. If we have family members going off to buy ice cream, I'll sometimes take my kids to buy a toy, shirt, or some other non-edible item. [9]

Disney Credit Card

I've had a Disney Chase credit card for years. I just switched to an American Airline credit card recently since we don't go to Disney as much now. But when we were going every year, it was nice because I always had a lot of "Disney Dollars" to spend at Disney. One year at Disney, I had $1,200 to spend! That was nice. We had no problem spending it all.

With your Disney Chase card, you get 10% off your purchases over $50 at the Disney stores. I got discounts on our Disney hotel stays sometimes too. You can get 10% off at some of the Disney hotel restaurants as well. Basically, if you are anywhere Disney, show them your Disney credit card and ask them if they offer the 10% discount there. [7]

Florida Resident Discounts

If you live in Florida, you probably already know that you can sometimes get a discount for being a Florida resident. My parents have a house in Florida so they can get a discount on Disney tickets for themselves and their grandkids (AKA - my kiddies!). For our Disney cruise, we also got a discount. They put one of my parents' names in each of our rooms so we would get a discount on both rooms. We did the same with our Disney hotel. The discount for the Disney hotel was only $25 but better than nothing. [8]

Perks When Staying at a Disney Hotel

When you're staying at a Disney hotel, you can have your purchases made at any other Disney location including the parks shipped back to your room for free. [9] For example, we bought some heavy dishes at Disney's Boardwalk and we were able to have those bags sent to our room and didn't have to carry them around with us all night. Just let the retail clerk know when you are checking out. They used to send your purchases to your hotel that same day but now they require at least 2 days to get your things back to your room.

Disney offers complimentary transportation from the airport to your Disney hotel on their Disney Magical Express buses. [10] You can also sometimes have your luggage picked up from the baggage claim at the airport and delivered to your room, as long as you travel on a participating airline. [11] Check with Disney at the time of your booking to arrange this. We had to put special tags on our luggage when we had the Disney Cruise Line pick up our luggage.

Keep in mind though that it can take up to 3 hours from your arrival time before your bags get delivered to your room.[11] I didn't realize this and we had to wait an hour or so for our bags before we could go swimming. So make sure to pack swim suits in your carry-on if you want to swim when you first get to the hotel.

Disney also offers transportation back to the airport from your hotel but make sure to arrange this the day before with the concierge. They can also hold your luggage and carry-on items for you right outside the front lobby if you want to walk around the hotel or eat breakfast before you catch your bus to the airport.

When staying at a Disney hotel, you also get free parking at the Disney parks during the length of your stay. You just need to show the parking attendant at the parks proof of your stay at a Disney hotel. Check with the front desk for more details. I didn't know this the last time we went! Could've saved us $20! [12]

You also get "Extra Magic Hours" at the parks when staying at a Disney hotel. Each day a different park is open extra hours for Disney resort guests. [13] For example, you may be able to get in to Magic Kingdom an hour before everyone else, or stay an hour later. Check your hotel concierge or Disney's online calendar for a list of parks, times, and details.

Shipping Items Home

You can have Disney mail your Disney store purchases to your home for you for a postage fee. We've done that. Make sure you keep your receipts in case you realize that you can't fit everything in your suitcase. They'll ask to see the receipt. Also, make sure you will be home by the time your package arrives, or ask a neighbor to stop by and pick up any packages left on your front porch before you arrive home. [9]

Chapter 9
Miscellaneous Items to Pack

Sunscreen

Don't forget the sunscreen! There are a few natural sunscreens that we like. All of them are very expensive (like $15-$20) so we try to just wear swim shirts, hats, or stay out of direct sunlight as much as possible. Luckily, my kids don't burn very easily. If we're going to be outside swimming all day or at the parks all day, we'll use sunscreen.

Our current favorite is the unscented 3rd Rock Sunblock. They have one variety that is "aromatherapeutic." We prefer the unscented. We've also used Goddess Garden Organics Sunny Kids and California Baby. California Baby goes on a little too thick for our liking. You can find these at your health food store, Whole Foods, or online. Ordering online from Amazon or Vitacost is usually cheaper than buying locally.

Owie Spray

Love this spray! We use it for everything! It's a mixture of lavender, tea tree oil, and frankincense, diluted with fractionated coconut oil (recipe at the end of the book). This is great for sunburn, mosquito bites, rashes, cuts, scrapes, bruises, bee stings, burns, acne - pretty much anything skin related. I bring it with in a sealed zip lock bag in my suitcase (no liquids over three ounces can go on the plane).

Epsom Salt

Epsom salt baths can be helpful if your child has a reaction. It helps the body detox and is calming.[1] Epsom salt is a source of magnesium as well. I always pack some Epsom salt in a zip lock bag and bring it in my suitcase.

We order our Epsom salt from San Francisco Salt Company online to ensure the salt is clean. We buy the 20 pound bag of Epsoak. Some Epsom salts have been rumored to contain metals and other contaminants. I'd rather be safe than sorry.

If you do buy your Epsom salts locally, make sure to at least get pharmaceutical grade Epsom salt. We use Epsom salt in every bath. We started with about ¼ cup and worked up to about 1 cup per bath. Small children can use ½ cup. As a general rule, you want to use about ½ cup per 50 pounds of weight. Have your child soak for at least 20 minutes. [1]

Towards the end of the bath you can also add some baking soda if you'd like. Baking soda helps absorb the toxins that the Epsom salt draws out. I just sprinkle some in. I probably only use about 1/8 of a cup but you can add up to 1 cup of baking soda. [1]

Some allergy moms will give their kids (over the age of 5) some baking soda (about ¼ to ½ of a teaspoon) mixed in with about 8 ounces of water, food, or some other drink like lemonade when their child is having a reaction to a food. [2]

Or some people make baking soda capsules by putting baking soda in to some empty veggie caps. The baking soda is an antacid that helps neutralize stomach acids in the stomach and can help alleviate an allergic reaction, especially if there is a respiratory reaction such as asthma or congestion or itchy eyes. [2]

Alka Seltzer Gold tablets can also be helpful for allergic reactions and work similar to the baking soda in neutralizing stomach acids. It makes the drink fizzy like a pop. [3]

Digestive Enzymes

We always take digestive enzymes when eating out as the chance of cross contamination is so high. For gluten and dairy, we use Houston Enzyme's AFP or Trienza. I prefer the AFP-Peptizyde as it contains a higher amount of the enzymes targeted for gluten and dairy. The Trienza includes AFP, Zyme Prime, and No Fenol in one. The Zyme Prime targets the digestion of carbs, and the No Fenol targets the digestion of phenols and salicylates. [4]

We used to use No Fenol enzymes to help deal with reactions and it seemed to help. It also seems to help some kids who accidentally (or intentionally) ingest food dyes. That's not to say that we can just take enzymes and not react like we normally would when eating these foods. It just aids in the digestion and can help lessen reactions.

Another benefit of No Fenol is that it breaks down the cell walls of yeast (Candida). Bonus. Just make sure your child is also taking some probiotics to help kill the yeast. For more information on how to take probiotics, visit my blog at www.allnaturalmomof4.com. I have a blog post entitled, "The Yeast Beast and Our Yeast Protocol." [5]

If you're using capsules, try to take the enzymes about 20 minutes before eating as it takes that long for the capsules to dissolve in your stomach. Houston Enzymes offers their enzymes in chewable form as well. You can contact them at 866-757-8627 to get free samples mailed to your house.

All of the Houston's chewables contain salicylates. As with anything, kids can react to digestive enzymes or one of the ingredients in the enzymes so try them out first before you decide to use them on vacation.

Other good digestive enzymes include Digest or Digest Gold by Enzymedica. You can order these enzymes online or sometimes you can find them at your local health food store or Whole Foods.

Homeopathics

If my kids get sick to their stomach, we use Nux Vomica (nice name, huh?) homeopathic pellets by Boiron. These contain a small amount of lactose (dairy) if your child is sensitive. For fevers, we use Belladonna. These are good to bring along with to the parks or on a cruise in case your kids get sick. We also take along Coldcalm for colds and Oscillococcinum for flu. You can find these at your local health food store.

Chapter 10
Resources for Disney Vacation Planning

Planning a Disney vacation takes hours! It's exhausting! One year I made a binder.

If you need help, I've used Larissa Boland at Custom Travel Professionals. You can find her on Facebook. She is also a Feingold mom so she is very familiar with food allergies and has some great tips for Disney!

It costs nothing extra to use a Disney travel professional. Disney takes care of them for bringing in the business. Larissa saved me a ton of time by emailing me prices for several different hotels so I could compare. Disney can look this up too but you spend a lot of time on the phone waiting for them to look up each hotel individually.

Web Sites

Sign up for some of the newsletters below prior to your trip to help you plan.

www.disneyparks.com (official Disney info)

www.disneydining.com (plan your dinner reservations) or call 407-WDW-DINE www.touringplans.com (info on best time to go, crowd expectations, etc.)

www.undercovertourist.com/orlando/crowd-calendar/ (crowd expectations, etc.)

www.mousesavers.com (discounts on Disney)

www.allergyfreemouse.com (great list of allergy free foods at Disney)

www.allergyeats.com/disney

www.glutenfreedairyfreewdw.com

www.gfinorlando.com

www.yourfirstvisit.net

www.disneyfanatic.com

www.mickeytips.com

www.howtodisney.com

www.disneylists.com

Books

The Unofficial Guide to Disney is a great book to check out from your library or purchase prior to your trip to help you plan.

Addresses for a Few Local Grocery Stores and Restaurants

(Below are close to Sea World and Universal Studios, near International Drive)

Whole Foods 8003 Turkey Lake Rd., Orlando

Trader Joe's 8323 W. Sand Lake Rd, Orlando

Chamberlin's Natural Health Food Store 7600 Dr. Phillips Blvd, Orlando

Five Guys 3042 W. Sand Lake Rd, Orlando

Chipotle 1700 W. Sand Lake Rd, Orlando

Panera Bread 7826 W. Sand Lake Rd, Orlando

There are several of the above restaurants throughout Orlando but only one Whole Foods.

If you have booked a Disney restaurant reservation (by calling 407-WDW-DINE), be sure to e-mail specialdiets@disneyworld.com at least 14 days ahead of time to discuss your dietary needs so they can be prepared for you when you arrive.

To book a Disney hotel reservation, call 407-939-1936 or contact a Disney travel agent.

Sample Meal Plan
(When you have a full kitchen)

Day 1:

Breakfast: Pancakes (Aunt Jemima or Namaste mix - freeze leftovers) and fruit

Lunch: Panera Bread

Dinner: Hamburgers or steak, baked potatoes or potato wedges, broccoli

Day 2:

Breakfast: Bacon, cereal or oatmeal, fruit

Lunch: Hot dogs, tomato or chicken and rice soup, sandwiches, and fruit for parks

Dinner: Eat at the parks

Day 3:

Breakfast: Smoothies, granola/protein bars, or bagels

Lunch: Chicken Tenders, green beans, watermelon

Dinner: Chipotle or another restaurant (steak perhaps)

Day 4:

Breakfast: Leftover pancakes or scrambled eggs, toast with jelly, fruit

Lunch: Grilled cheese, tater tots, peas, fruit, or Annie's mac-n-cheese

Dinner: Spaghetti, salad, and asparagus

Day 5:

Breakfast: Smoothies and donuts from Erin's Bakery (at Disney Springs)

Lunch: Five Guys Burgers and Fries

Dinner: Garlic lime chicken and rice, green beans

Day 6:

Breakfast: Cereal, oatmeal, fruit, or leftovers

Lunch: Tacos with corn chips, lettuce, and tomato. Chips and salsa.

Dinner: Order Papa John's Pizza

Day 7:

Breakfast: Eat all the leftovers!

Lunch: Pack a lunch for the plane ride home - sandwiches, fruit, snacks

Dinner: Panera Bread or Chipotle

Snacks:

> Microwave popcorn, So Delicious ice cream and ice cream
> bars, soup, Boom Chicka Pop popcorn

Obviously, adjust this to your family's likes and your schedule for the week. This is just a sample to provide some ideas to help you get started with your planning. Our family has members with different food allergies. Please do your own research to determine which foods are suitable for your family's dietary needs.

I left some blank pages at the end of the book for you to make your own meal plan and shopping list if you'd like.

Sample Shopping List
(When you have a full kitchen)

You don't have to get all your groceries at once if you are close to the Whole Foods or you have a car. And remember to save your receipts. My kids often eat four meals a day so you'll see some processed foods below that are not included in the meal plan. This is also for those picky kids who don't always eat what everyone else is eating!

Shopping List – Whole Foods

Steak, chicken breasts, ground beef

Applegate farms beef hot dogs

Organic eggs

Rudi's Honey Sweet Whole Wheat bread

Rudi's GF bread

Strawberry jelly (any organic)

Ian's chicken nugget meal (GF)

Bell & Evans GF chicken tenders

Pacific Original rice milk

Organic milk

365 organic green beans - frozen

365 organic peas - frozen

365 organic tater tots

365 frozen blueberries

365 frozen raspberries

365 frozen strawberries

So Delicious Salted Caramel Cluster cashew milk ice cream

So Delicious Mocha Almond Fudge almond milk ice cream bars

Julie's ice cream sandwiches (not dairy free)

365 organic rotini noodles

Gluten free Tinkyada brown rice spaghetti noodles

Annie's mac-n-cheese

Spaghetti sauce (Muir Glen, etc.)

Olive oil (small bottle)

Daiya cheddar cheese shreds

Horizon organic cheese

Earth Balance butter – soy free, red container or Horizon Organic butter

Natural by Nature whip cream

Maple syrup – small bottle

Imagine creamy tomato soup

Pacific organic chicken broth

Pacific chicken and rice soup

Glutino crackers – original (for tomato soup)

Kinnikinnick graham crackers (GFCF)

Dandies marshmallows

Namaste GFCF pancake and waffle mix

Late July corn chips

Kind bars, Nugo chocolate protein bars, etc.

Organic romaine lettuce

Salad dressing (Marie's Creamy Italian or Follow Your Heart Dairy Free Ranch)

Cucumber

Fruit –organic apples, strawberries, red grapes, oranges, grapefruit, cantaloupe, watermelon, bananas, etc.

White organic potatoes (bag)

Tomatoes

2 limes (for the garlic lime chicken)

Fresh broccoli

Fresh asparagus

365 pop – Root beer

Publix or Wal-Mart: (located across from the Whole Foods)

Hormel turkey slices – Oven Roasted

Bacon (Hormel Natural) If they don't have Hormel, get Applegate Farms from Whole Foods

Ketchup – Hunt's All Natural "No Corn Syrup Added"

Water bottles (Fiji)

Simply Lemonade, or lemons and sugar to make lemonade

Aunt Jemima pancake mix (Original not the "Complete")

Food To Bring from Home

Cereal (individual serving sizes in quart size freezer bags. Envirokids, etc.)

Taco seasoning

Garlic lime chicken seasoning

Salt and pepper for potato wedges

Chicken nugget seasoning

2 cups of organic rice

Oatmeal packets (Glutenfreeda Apple Cinnamon)

Cinnamon for oatmeal

Popcorn for microwave

Snacks for plane

Few chocolate granola bars for the backpack cooler

Aunt Jemima pancake mix in a zip lock bag (in case you can't find any in Florida)

Protein powder for smoothies (we use Sunwarrior Vanilla and Vega Protein and Greens Berry flavored)

Individual small Cracker Barrel syrups if you don't want to buy maple syrup in Florida.

When we go to Cracker Barrel, I always save any extra unopened syrups and use them for vacation or send them with my son to camp.

Sample Meal Suggestions
(Without a full kitchen)

Breakfasts: Fruit, bagels (Einstein Bagels, Panera Bread, or Whole Foods), cereal, oatmeal, granola bars, protein bars, Kind bars, 365 beef jerky or organic beef sticks, donuts from Erin's Bakery in Disney Springs, smoothies (if you bring a blender), premade muffins and pancakes from home (if you drove your car there), or eat out at a Disney restaurant, Starbuck's, or Cracker Barrel.

Lunches: Annie's microwavable mac-n-cheese, Ian's chicken nugget microwavable meals, Amy's microwavable meals like Baked Ziti, sandwiches, deli meat, summer sausage, cheese, and crackers, salad, canned peaches or pears, baby carrots and Marie's Creamy Ranch dressing, or eat out.

Dinners: Eat out at a Disney hotel or restaurant, Five Guys, Chipotle, Panera Bread, Olive Garden, Subway, McDonald's, Wendy's, or order Papa John's Pizza.

Snacks: Microwave popcorn, s'mores (Dandies marshmallows, graham crackers from Whole Foods, and Enjoy Life or Ghirardelli chocolate chips), Late July corn chips and Muir Glen salsa, chips and fresh guacamole from Whole Foods, or fruit. For dessert, So Delicious ice cream and ice cream bars (leave in the hotel's freezer if staying at a Disney hotel).

If you're staying in a regular hotel, you'll likely be eating out for most of your meals. Breakfast and snacks are pretty easy to do at the hotel. For lunch and dinner, we typically eat out unless we drove and we're only staying for a couple of days. Then I'm able to bring more food from home.

Sample Shopping List
(Without a full kitchen)

Shopping List – Whole Foods

Rudi's Honey Sweet Whole Wheat bread

Deli meats

Ian's chicken nugget meal (GF) - leave in hotel freezer

Amy's GFCF Baked Ziti (microwavable meal) - leave in hotel freezer

Pacific Original rice milk or regular organic milk

365 frozen blueberries (if doing smoothies)

365 frozen raspberries (if doing smoothies)

365 frozen strawberries (if doing smoothies)

So Delicious Salted Caramel Cluster cashew milk ice cream - leave in hotel freezer

So Delicious Mocha Almond Fudge almond milk ice cream bars - leave in hotel freezer

Annie's microwavable mac-n-cheese packets (or bring from home)

Kinnikinnick graham crackers (GFCF)

Dandies marshmallows

Late July corn chips

Muir Glen salsa

Fresh made guacamole (near produce)

Kind bars, Nugo chocolate protein bars, etc.

Organic romaine lettuce

Salad dressing (Marie's Creamy Italian or Follow Your Heart Dairy Free Ranch)

Cucumber

Fruit –organic apples, strawberries, grapes, oranges, grapefruit, cantaloupe, watermelon, bananas, etc.

365 pop – Root beer

Publix or Wal-Mart: (located across from the Whole Foods)

Hormel turkey slices – Oven Roasted

Ketchup – Hunt's All Natural "No Corn Syrup Added" (or get some ketchup packets from a restaurant. Will have corn syrup.)

Water bottles (Fiji or other)

Simply Lemonade (individual bottles for parks)

To Bring from Home

Cereal (individual serving sizes in quart size freezer bags. Envirokids, etc.)

Oatmeal packets (Glutenfreeda Apple Cinnamon)

Cinnamon for oatmeal

Popcorn for microwave

Snacks for plane

Few chocolate granola bars for the back pack cooler

Protein powder for smoothies (we use Sunwarrior Vanilla and Vega Protein and Greens Berry flavored)

Other Items to Pack

Probiotics

Vitamins (I use pill boxes I got on Amazon)

Digestive enzymes

Epsom salt

Books to read

New toys, coloring books, stickers, games, for the plane ride (don't show the kids yet!)

I-Pod and headphones

I-Pads and headphones for the kids

Any recipes needed

Plane tickets/boarding passes (check in online the night before)

Rental car receipt/confirmation

Insulated food thermoses

Ceramic bowl and spoon

Tupperware for the parks

Sports bottles for the parks (pack in suitcase)

Lunch for the plane ride

Snacks for the plane

Gum for the plane

Sunglasses

Hats

Sunscreen

Phone and tablet chargers

Car charger

Candy (gummy worms, fruit chews, etc.)

Car seat

Stroller

Recipes

Chicken Nuggets

3 cups of rice cereal (Erewhon, Barbara's, etc.)
2 TB flour
1 tsp dried thyme
1 tsp dried sage
1 tsp sugar (I use organic sugar from Costco)
½ tsp paprika (omit for stage one)
½ tsp salt (I use Redmond's Real Sea Salt)
½ tsp pepper
½ cup olive oil
4 boneless chicken breasts

Preheat oven to 400 degrees. Combine the dry ingredients in a food processor or blender. Place a portion of the crumb mixture in a shallow bowl. (I put at least half of the crumb mixture into a zip lock freezer bag and save for later use.) In another bowl, put the oil. Cut chicken into chicken nugget size cubes. Dip chicken in oil, then in crumb mixture.

Place nuggets on a pan lined with unbleached parchment paper (from WF) that has been brushed lightly with oil. Bake at 400 degrees for 20-22 minutes until cooked through.

I double the above recipe and keep the crumb mixture in a mason quart jar to save time when I am making chicken nuggets. These are a staple in our house.

*Adapted from a recipe from "Special Eats" by Sueson Vess.

Feingold Stage 2 (for stage 1, omit the paprika)

Chicken Tenders

I adapted this recipe from our favorite GFCF (gluten and dairy free) cookbook called "Cooking for Isaiah" by Silvana Nardone.

6 cups Fritos or other corn chips crushed (I throw mine in my food processor)
1 tsp salt (or less to taste - I use ½ tsp because the chips are already salty)
½ tsp pepper
3 eggs (I use organic olive oil instead.)

Cut up chicken breasts into strips then dip chicken into a small bowl of olive oil (or slightly beaten eggs if you can do eggs). Coat chicken with corn chip mixture and place on to a slightly oiled baking dish. Cook at 425 degrees for 20-25 minutes.

I use the Frito Scoops for this recipe. Fritos have cross contamination issues but the Scoops are supposed to be run on a separate line so have less CC issues if you have a gluten sensitivity. Everyone really likes these. (Frito Lay will no longer work with Feingold but used to be approved for years. We still use them without a problem.)

Some kids like to dip the chicken tenders in ranch dressing like Marie's Creamy Italian.

Feingold Stage 1

Garlic Lime Chicken and Rice

1 tsp salt (I use sea salt)

½ to 1 tsp pepper (I use ½ for lower oxalate, but recipe calls for 1)

1 tsp garlic powder

½ tsp onion powder

½ tsp thyme

¼ tsp paprika (omit for stage 1)

¼ tsp cayenne pepper (omit for stage 1)

2 TB butter

2 TB olive oil (I use organic)

½ cup chicken broth (I use organic Pacific brand)

4 TB fresh lime juice

4 boneless skinless chicken breasts (about 1 lb)

In a bowl, mix together the seasonings. Sprinkle mixture onto both sides of the chicken breasts. I use about ¼ tsp of the seasonings on each side of a large organic chicken breast. How much you use depends on how spicy you want it. I like it spicier, but then my kids won't eat it. About 1/4 tsp on each side seems to work.

In a skillet, heat butter and oil over medium high heat. Sauté chicken until golden brown and cooked through, about 5-7 minutes on each side. Turn down the heat and remove chicken and keep warm (put a plate over them). Add the lime juice and chicken broth to the pan until heated through. Add chicken back to the pan and serve. I like to serve with rice and drizzle some of the lime juice mixture over it. I double the above recipe, and keep the seasonings in a jar for when I make this. We make this often.

*Adapted from a recipe on www.flylady.com.

Feingold Stage 2 (stage 1 if you omit the paprika and cayenne pepper)

Hamburger/Steak Seasoning

2TB Kosher salt
1 TB pepper
½ TB garlic salt
½ TB onion salt
1 tsp celery salt

Combine all ingredients and store in a small glass jar. Right before cooking, sprinkle the seasoning over hamburgers or steaks on one side only. This is the seasoning they use at *Cheeseburger in Paradise* restaurants.

We use Rudi's Organic Whole Wheat buns from Trader Joe's or Whole Foods. Or King's Hawaiian hamburger buns (some kids have issues with these though).

Feingold Stage 1

Taco Seasoning

Stage 1 Recipe:

1 tsp onion powder

1 tsp salt

½ tsp pepper

¼ tsp garlic powder

¼ tsp oregano

1 ½ tsp ground cumin

½ tsp tapioca or corn starch as a thickener

Stage 2 Recipe: (This is what we use)

2 tsp onion powder

1 tsp chili powder

½ tsp crushed red pepper

¼ tsp dried oregano

1 tsp salt

½ tsp tapioca starch (you could also use organic corn starch)

½ tsp garlic powder

½ tsp ground cumin

Combine all ingredients. I double or triple the above recipe and keep stored in a small glass jar. I use 2 tsp for 1 lb of meat because my kids do not like it spicy. Adjust to taste.

Potato Wedges

My mom makes these for holidays and everyone always asks her for the recipe. She just laughs. It's very simple!

6 organic russet or other white potatoes (about 1 per person)
1/8 to ¼ cup of olive oil
1 tsp salt
About 10 twists of fresh ground pepper (or about 1/2 tsp of pepper)

Wash potatoes thoroughly. You can peel the potato skins or leave them on. I usually leave them on.

Cut the potatoes in half lengthwise, and then one more time. (Depending on how big the potatoes are, I'll cut them in fourths or eighths.) Place potatoes in a 9x13 baking dish and sprinkle with enough olive oil to lightly cover the potatoes. Mix until all the potatoes are covered in oil. Sprinkle with the salt and pepper. If you can do stage two, you can add about ½ tsp each of paprika and chili powder as well.

Place on a pan with sides (this is best as the darker pan will help get the potatoes brown and crisp), or I've been just using a glass 9x13 baking dish. It's best not to let the potatoes touch too much or they will end up soggy instead of crisp. Bake at 425 degrees for 45 minutes, or until tender and lightly browned. I flip the potatoes halfway through cooking.

Feingold Stage 1

Chocolate Granola Bars

These are good right out of the freezer too. They defrost quickly. I like that they contain a lot of oats. Oats have a calming effect.

3/4 cup (1 1/2 sticks) butter, softened
1/3 cup brown sugar, packed (Domino brand)
1 tsp vanilla extract
1 cup whole wheat flour (regular flour is probably fine too)
1 tsp baking soda
1 TB ground flax seed (optional)
4 1/2 cups rolled oats
1 cup (6 ounces) semi-sweet chocolate chips (I use Ghirardelli)

Instructions:

Preheat oven to 325 degrees. In a medium-size mixing bowl, cream together the butter, honey, brown sugar, and vanilla extract. (I used an electric mixer.)

Add flour, baking soda, and oats. Stir until well-mixed. Stir in chocolate chips. Using a spatula, press mixture into a lightly-greased (I use coconut oil) 9x13-inch baking dish. Bake at 325 degrees for 18-22 minutes, until edges are just starting to brown. Remove from oven and place dish on wire rack to cool.

Cool granola bars, and then cut with a sharp knife. I store these in the freezer in a large zip lock bag. They defrost quickly.

Feingold Stage 1

Rice Krispy Treats

5 cups of rice krispy cereal (we use Erewhon)
2 TB of butter (we use Earth Balance soy free buttery spread)
2 TB coconut oil (or use all butter)
1 package of Dandie's marshmallows (these contain soy)

Directions:

Melt butter, coconut oil, and marshmallows over low heat, stirring the entire time. It takes a little while for the marshmallows to melt. Add the rice krispies and stir to combine. Transfer to an 8x11 pan. Use cookie cutters to cut out into shapes if desired. These will start to get hard after a day or two.

Feingold Stage 1

Sugar Cookies

½ cup butter, softened (try to let the butter sit out for half hour before using)

1 cup sugar

1 egg (bring to room temp by placing in a bowl of warm water)

1 TB lemon juice (I use fresh squeezed)

1 tsp vanilla (watch for corn syrup)

2 cups flour (any is fine but I like King Arthur unbleached)

½ tsp salt

½ tsp baking soda

1. Cream butter and sugar until light and fluffy.
2. Beat in egg, lemon juice, and vanilla.
3. Combine dry ingredients, and gradually beat into the butter mixture until well blended.
4. Divide dough into two balls and flatten to 1-inch thickness.
5. Wrap in plastic wrap. Refrigerate at least 2 hours or overnight.

Preheat oven to 375. Roll out dough onto floured surface. To reduce sticking, use some wax paper to put over top the dough and roll to 1/8 to ¼ thickness. Remove wax paper and cut with cookie cutters.

Place on an ungreased cookie sheet leaving 1 inch between cookies. Bake 8-12 minutes (depending on size of cookie, thickness, and the pan you are using). I do about 9 minutes. Cool on a rack.

Decorate with cookie frosting and sugar crystals (optional). I get India Tree sugar crystals from Whole Foods or you can order online.

<u>Cookie Frosting</u>
2 ¼ cup powdered sugar
2 ½ TB vegetable oil (I use canola oil)
2 ½ TB water
¼ tsp vanilla
Pinch of salt

<u>Here's another frosting recipe:</u>
3 1/8 cups powdered sugar
1 TB canola oil
1 TB butter, melted
1 TB milk
1 TB water, and a pinch of salt
½ tsp. vanilla

Beat all ingredients together. Add more water to get the proper consistency.

If you want to color the frosting, you can use India Tree or Confection Crafts natural food dyes.

Feingold Stage 1

Ant Killer Spray

10 drops of tea tree oil

5 drops of lavender

5 drops of lemon or lemongrass

5 drops of eucalyptus (omit if you have young kids)

5 drops of peppermint

2 TB of fractionated coconut oil

1 TB of witch hazel (keeps oils dispersed)

Combine all of the above in a small glass or amber colored spray bottle and shake to combine. I double the above recipe when I make it. Be careful when spraying essential oils. Oils like peppermint and eucalyptus can cause breathing issues in infants and young kids or dogs. I try to spray at night or right before we leave for vacation.

It does leave an oily residue but I just wipe it up later. It works well to keep the ants away for a few days. Sometimes I'll just throw some water, olive oil, and a few drops of peppermint oil into a spray bottle as well if I'm being lazy. That works too.

Owie Spray

4 TB fractionated coconut oil
5 drops of lavender
5 drops of tea tree oil (melaleuca)
5 drops of frankincense

Combine in a small glass spray bottle. I got one at my local health food store or you can order online at places like www.bulkapothecary.com. This is where I ordered my fractionated coconut oil. Fractionated coconut oil is used because it stays in a liquid state, unlike regular coconut oil which hardens at cooler temperatures. Can double the above recipe if desired.

Shake and use on mosquito bites, sunburn, cuts, bruises, bee stings, acne, rashes, or burns. It's best not to use on open wounds (though we have) but once the wound is no longer exposed, spray on the area 2 to 3 times per day. This works great! My kids ask for it any time they get hurt.

Meal Plan

Day 1:

    <u>Breakfast:</u>

    <u>Lunch:</u>

    <u>Dinner:</u>

Day 2:

    <u>Breakfast:</u>

    <u>Lunch:</u>

    <u>Dinner:</u>

Day 3:

    <u>Breakfast:</u>

    <u>Lunch:</u>

    <u>Dinner:</u>

Day 4:

Breakfast:

Lunch:

Dinner:

Day 5:

Breakfast:

Lunch:

Dinner:

Day 6:

Breakfast:

Lunch:

Dinner:

Day 7:

Breakfast:

Lunch:

Dinner:

Snacks:

Shopping List

Whole Foods

Shopping List

Publix or Wal-Mart:
(located across from the Whole Foods)

To Bring from Home

Other Items to Pack

Check out Sheri Davis' first book, *"All Natural Mom's Guide to the Feingold Diet"* available on Amazon for more information on how to treat ADHD naturally and avoid dyes and artificial ingredients. Visit her blog at www.allnaturalmomof4.com.

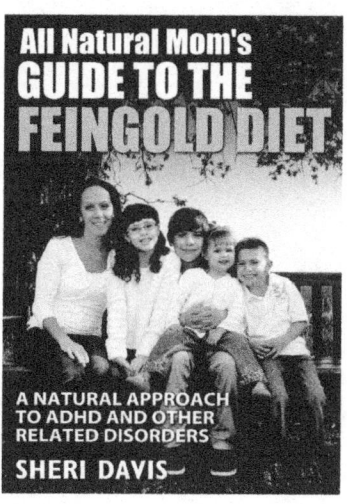

And coming soon! *"Living Dye Free in a Cotton Candy World"* will cover the practical implementation of a diet free of dyes, artificial flavors, and preservatives. How does one deal with class parties, Halloween, vacations, birthdays, illnesses, doctor visits, and unsupportive relatives? Sheri Davis covers it all in this must-read, information-packed book!

About the Author

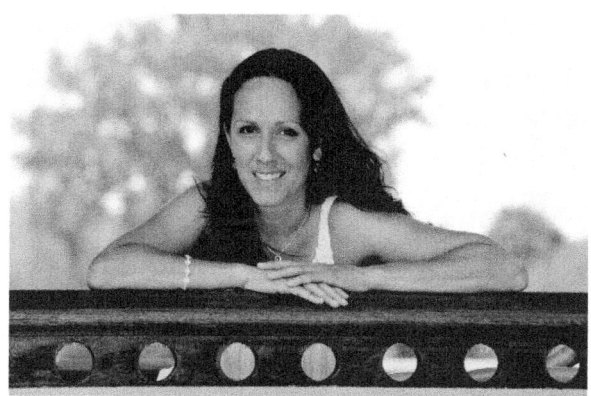

Sheri Davis is the mother of four kids between the ages of 6 and 16. She is the author of the book, *"All Natural Mom's Guide to the Feingold Diet - A Natural Approach to ADHD and Other Related Disorders."*

Sheri is an ADHD Diet and Biomed Coach and blogs and speaks on the Feingold Diet, the GFCF diet, supplements, biomed, her faith, and all things natural at www.allnaturalmomof4.com. Sheri loves helping parents help their kids.

Sheri and her family reside in northern Illinois. She has a Bachelor's degree in Business Administration from Elmhurst College.

You can also find her on Facebook at
www.facebook.com/allnaturalmom.

References

Introduction

1. Davis, Sheri. "What Is the Feingold Diet?" 12/22/14. www.allnaturalmomof4.com. Accessed at http://www.allnaturalmomof4.com/2014/12/what-is-feingold-die.html.
2. "Epsom Salts." 08/25/05. www.enzymestuff.com. Accessed at http://www.enzymestuff.com/epsomsalts.htm.

Chapter 1

1. "5 Reasons to LOVE Garden Grocer Delivery Service." 01/21/17. www.chipandco.com. Accessed at http://www.chipandco.com/5-reasons-love-garden-grocer-delivery-service-2-99045/.
2. "8 Ways to Get Groceries at Disney World." 09/10/16. www.wdwprepschool.com. Accessed at http://wdwprepschool.com/8-ways-to-get-groceries-at-disney-world/.
3. Bricker, Tom. "Tips for Using Uber at Disney World." (n.d.). www.disneytouristblog.com. Accessed at http://www.disneytouristblog.com/uber-disney-world-tips/.

Chapter 2

1. "Summary of the HIPAA Privacy Rule." (n.d.). www.hhs.gov. Accessed at http://www.hhs.gov/hipaa/for-professionals/privacy/laws-regulations/.
2. Bomkamp, Samantha. "McDonald's, In a Bid To Woo Health-Focused Diners, Will Remove Some Artificial Preservatives." 08/01/16. www.chicagotribune.com. Accessed at http://www.chicagotribune.com/business/ct-mcdonalds-food-0802-biz-20160801-story.html.

Chapter 5

1. Horovitz, Bruce. "Chipotle: GMO's Gone From Our Food." 04/27/15. Accessed at http://www.usatoday.com/story/money/2015/04/27/chipotle-fast-food-restaurants-gmos-genetically-modified-ingredents/26450061/.
2. Lowin, Rebekah. "Chipotle Now Boasts Zero Preservatives - And a New Tortilla." 03/28/17. www.foodandwine.com. Accessed at http://www.foodandwine.com/news/chipotle-rebrands.
3. Bomkamp, Samantha. "McDonald's, In a Bid To Woo Health-Focused Diners, Will Remove Some Artificial Preservatives." 08/01/16. www.chicagotribune.com. Accessed at http://www.chicagotribune.com/business/ct-mcdonalds-food-0802-biz-20160801-story.html
4. "Panera Bread to Remove Artificial Additives From the Menu by 2016." 06/04/14. www.foxnews.com. Accessed at http://www.foxnews.com/health/2014/06/04/panera-

bread-to-remove-artificial-additives-from-menu-by-2016.html.

5. Davis, Sheri. "Papa John's Pizza." 01/19/13. www.allnaturalmomof4.com. Accessed at http://theallnaturaldiet.blogspot.com/2013/01/papa-johns-pizza.html.

6. Gelski, Jeff. "Papa John's Completes Removal of 14 Ingredients." 10/4/16. www.foodbusinessnews.net. Accessed at http://www.foodbusinessnews.net/articles/news_home/Food-Service-Retail/2016/10/Papa_Johns_completes_removal_o.aspx?ID=%7B4F4FDAC5-2251-419D-ACAE-B265515147D3%7D&cck=1.

7. "Better Ingredients." www.papajohns.com. Accessed at http://www.papajohns.com/company/papa-johns-ingredients.html#sauces.

8. "Explore Our Menu." (n.d.). www.starbucks.com. Accessed at http://www.starbucks.com/menu/catalog/product?food=bakery#view_control=product.

9. Daniela, Garlaza. "Subway Will Drop Artificial Ingredients by 2017." 06/04/15. www.eater.com. Accessed at http://www.eater.com/2015/6/4/8727495/subway-will-drop-artificial-ingredients-by-2017.

10. "Wendy's "Natural Cut" Fries. Indeed?" 04/17/11. www.fooducate.com. Accessed at http://www.fooducate.com/app#!page=post&id=57A339ED-8648-0337-4A6F-96713D6CA84D.

Chapter 6

1. "Guests With Disabilities." (n.d.). www.sixflags.com. Accessed at http://www.sixflags.com/greatamerica/plan-your-visit/guests-with-disabilities.
2. "Galactic Grill Allergy Friendly Lunch and Dinner Menu." 12/29/16. www.glutenfreedairyfreewdw.com. Accessed at http://www.glutenfreedairyfreewdw.com/galactic-grill-allergy-friendly-lunch-dinner-menu/.
3. "Cosmic Ray's Allergy Friendly Lunch and Dinner Menu." 10/27/15. www.glutenfreedairyfreewdw.com. Accessed at http://www.glutenfreedairyfreewdw.com/cosmic-rays-allergy-friendly-lunch-and-dinner-menu/.
4. "Gluten Free Dining at Disney." (n.d.). www.diningatdisney.com. Accessed at http://diningatdisney.com/gluten-free-dining-at-disney/.
5. "Fairytale Dining Dinner at Cinderella's Royal Table - Magic Kingdom." 04/11/16. www.gfinorlando.com. Accessed at http://www.gfinorlando.com/2016/04/fairytale-dining-dinner-at-cinderellas.html.
6. "Liberty Tree Tavern -Dinner - Table Service - Magic Kingdom." 11/08/13. www.glutenfreedairyfreewdw.com. Accessed at http://www.glutenfreedairyfreewdw.com/liberty-tree-tavern-dinner-table-service-magic-kingdom/.
7. "Tony's Town Square Guest Post Food Allergy Review." (n.d.). www.allergyfreemouse.com. Accessed at http://www.allergyfreemouse.com/2012/02/tonys-town-square-guest-post-food-allergy-review/.

8. "Peco's Bill Tall Tale Inn and Café - Magic Kingdom."
    09/12/15. www.gfinorlando.com. Accessed at
    http://www.gfinorlando.com/2015/09/pecos-bill-tall-tale-
    inn-and-cafe-magic.html.
9. "Walkers Shortbread Mickey Mouse Cookies." (n.d.).
    www.disneyworld.disneylandfloralandgifts.com. Accessed
    at
    http://disneyworld.disneyfloralandgifts.com/product/walke
    rs-shortbread-mickey-mouse-cookies-4.4-oz.do.

Chapter 8

1. "Orlando Crowd Calendar." (n.d.).
    www.undercovertourist.com. Accessed at
    http://www.undercovertourist.com/orlando/crowd-
    calendar/
2. www.touringplan.com. (n.d.). Accessed at
    http://touringplans.com/walt-disney-world/events/gay-
    days.
3. Sietzer, Jana. "Allergy-Friendly Mickey's Not So Scary
    Halloween Party." 04/06/17. www.travelingmom.com.
    Accessed at http://www.travelingmom.com/top-
    destinations-disney/allergy-friendly-mickeys-not-so-scary-
    halloween-party/.
4. www.wdw.info.com. (n.d.). Accessed at
    http://www.wdwinfo.com/wdwinfo/fastpass.htm.
5. "Guests With Disabilities - Frequently Asked Questions."
    www.disneyworld.disney.go.com. (n.d.). Accessed at
    http://disneyworld.disney.go.com/faq/guests-with-
    disabilities/attraction-access/.

6. "Guests With Disabilities." (n.d.). www.sixflags.com. Accessed at http://www.sixflags.com/greatamerica/plan-your-visit/guests-with-disabilities.

7. www.disneyrewards.com. (n.d.). Accessed at http://disneyrewards.com/walt-disney-world-perks/.

8. "Special Florida Resident Tickets and Passes." (n.d.). www.disneyworld.disney.go.com. Accessed at http://disneyworld.disney.go.com/florida-residents/.

9. "Package Pickup." (n.d.). www.disneyworld.disney.go.com. Accessed at http://disneyworld.disney.go.com/guest-services/package-pickup-and-delivery/.

10. "Airport Transportation and Check In." (n.d.). www.disneyworld.disney.go.com. Accessed at http://disneyworld.disney.go.com/faq/airport-transportation-and-check-in/magical-express-costs/.

11. "Airport Transportation and Check In." (n.d.). Accessed at http://disneyworld.disney.go.com/faq/airport-transportation-and-check-in/luggage-delivery/.

12. "Why Stay at a Disney Resort Hotel?" (n.d.). www.disneyworld.disney.go.com. Accessed at http://disneyworld.disney.go.com/resort-hotels-benefits/#/drawer=drawerComplimentaryTransportation.

13. "Why Stay at a Disney Resort Hotel?" (n.d.). www.disneyworld.disney.go.com. Accessed at https://disneyworld.disney.go.com/guest-services/extra-magic-hours/.

Chapter 9

1. Jockers, David, Dr. "Benefits of Epsom Salt Baths - A Powerful (And Cheap!) Detoxifier." (n.d.). www.thetruthaboutcancer.com. Accessed at http://thetruthaboutcancer.com/benefits-epsom-salt-baths/.
2. Bright, Sierra. "5 Reasons You Should Try Drinking Baking Soda." 1/15/16. www.naturallivingideas.com. Accessed at http://www.naturallivingideas.com/drinking-baking-soda-benefits/.
3. Williams, David, Dr. "My Natural Treatments and Remedies for Food Allergies and Food Intolerances." (n.d.). www.drdavidwilliams.com. http://www.drdavidwilliams.com/food-allergies-natural-treatments.
4. "Frequently Asked Questions." (n.d.). http://www.houston-enzymes.com Accessed at https://www.houston-enzymes.com/learn/faq.php.
5. Davis, Sheri. "The Yeast Beast and Our Yeast Protocol." 05/01/13. www.allnaturalmomof4.com. Accessed at http://www.allnaturalmomof4.com/2013/05/the-yeast-beast-and-our-yeast-protoco.html.

Made in the USA
Monee, IL
07 July 2026

56552274R00075